DEDICATION

This book is dedicated to my favorite ex-Valspeaker, who sought to improve her "total image" and succeeded—Deborah Zafman.

ACKNOWLEDGMENTS

The authors wish to convey their *total* appreciation to Peter Workman and the hardworking people who helped us in making this book: our editor, Suzanne Rafer; our copy editor, Louise Gikow; our art director, Paul Hanson; our photographer, Robin Holland; and our stylists, Becky Sangster and Linda Choe.

We are *fully* indebted to our models: cover girl Zoë Weaver; Genevieve Anderson; Deborah Gahr; Jessica Gerson; Sara Martin; Susan Randall; Vanessa Southern; Kyle Thomes; and Eric Hernandez, a vicious Dude.

Our special thanks goes to Professor Peter Ladefoged and Dr. Hector Javkin of the Speech Laboratory at UCLA for providing what may be the world's first visual records of Valspeak; Dr. June E. Shoup, Chairman of the Department of Communication, Arts and Sciences, and the Speech Communication Research Laboratory at the University of Southern California; KABC-TV/Eyewitness News for the successful Valley Girl segment and also for their encouragement and support, especially that of Dennis Swanson, Terry Crowfoot, Ken Nelson, Jim Hattendorf, Charles Darling, Maggie Simms, Pat Higgins, Vic Heman, Millie Martinez, Art Gluskoter, Jim Myrah, Maureen Conners, and the entire staff and crew—no wonder KABC is the number one station; Marc Davidson of the University of Southern California Press Services for his support, insight and wit; the American Speech, Language, and Hearing Association and the National Association for Hearing and Speech Action; and finally, thanks to Sid Graw for his constant encouragement and confidence.

HOW TO DEPROGRAM YOUR VALLEY GIRL

BY DR. LILLIAN GLASS

With Richard Liebmann-Smith

Photographs by Robin Holland

A LIGHTNING BOOK

from Workman Publishing, New York

Published simultaneously in Canada by Saunders of Toronto, Inc.

Library of Congress Cataloging in Publication Data

Glass, Lillian.
How to deprogram your valley girl

1. English language—Anecdotes, facetiae, satire, etc.
2. Youth—Language (New words, slang, etc.)—Anecdotes, facetiae, satire, etc. I. Liebmann-Smith, Richard.
II. Title.
PN6231.D6G5 1982 427'.97949'0207 82-21964
ISBN 0-89480-239-9

Cover and book design: Paul Hanson
Cover and book photographs: Robin Holland
Cover cosmetician: Grace Maltese

Photo Credits

FLAPPER: The Bettmann Archive
BOBBY SOXER: United Press International Photo
HIPPIE: Roger Malloch, Magnum

Workman Publishing Company, Inc.
1 West 39th Street
New York, NY 10018

A Lightning Book
Manufactured in the United States of America
First printing December 1982
10 9 8 7 6 5 4 3 2 1

CONTENTS

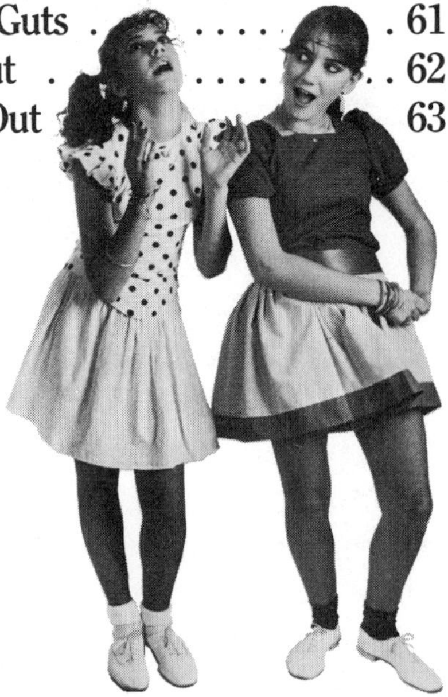

INTRODUCTION

INVASION OF THE VALLEY PEOPLE

Not long ago, I began receiving an unusually high number of telephone calls from parents requesting speech and communication therapy for their teenagers. At first I thought that well-meaning parents wanted to see their sons and daughters better their "total communication image" during their summer vacation. But as more and more arrived at my office, I noticed that there was a high percentage of clients—male and female—who all seemed to sound alike, and I wondered if indeed this might be some rare syndrome affecting California teenagers of both sexes.

One day while in my car, I turned on the radio and heard a familiar sound. A song called "Valley Girl" was playing. I couldn't believe my ears: Moon Unit Zappa's characterization of a Valley Girl sounded just like my clients. That night during the communications class I teach at U.S.C., I began listening more closely to my juniors and seniors and found the same speech pattern developing there as well.

Based on these incidents, I decided to cover the "Valley" sound in a segment on my weekly medical and communication report on KABC-TV/Eyewitness News in Los Angeles. The response was overwhelming. The wire services picked up the story and the next thing I knew, I was swamped with radio, TV, newspaper, and magazine interviews on how I "deprogram" Valspeakers. The Valspeak phenomenon, it seems, was not limited to the San Fernando Valley in California. People all over the United States and Canada seemed to be speaking this peculiar "language."

But the words of Valspeak are not the only problem. Each generation always has its own slang vocabulary. Only ten years ago mine used words and phrases like "far out," "hip," "groovy," and "do your own thing." The phenomenon of Valspeak seemed more alarming to me, though, not only because parents were dissatisfied with the way their sons and daughters were speaking, but because they seemed to be doing so while excluding all other communication elements. In other words, not only was there a substitution of slang for meaningful dialogue, but there was also a monotone quality in speaking, a rapid rate of speaking, lack of proper breath control, excessive nasality, abnormal pitch, and constant repetition of words and phrases.

My doctoral research had shown that the way a person speaks is of greater importance than the way that person looks. Think of the billions of dollars we spend on the latest fashions, hairstyles, makeup, and diet plans. What about spending some time on the way we talk? We communicate during 80 percent of our waking day; how many of us do it well? This book is designed—in a humorous way—to enable parents and their Vals to communicate better.

Dr. Lillian Glass

IS THERE A VAL IN THE HOUSE?

Every twenty years, it seems, something happens in America that produces a new strain of youth. In the 1920s we had the Flapper. Her hair was bobbed, her knees were bare, she danced the Charleston to hot jazz and said, "Oh you kid." Two decades later the Bobby Soxer came on the scene. She wore tight sweaters, saddle shoes, danced the Lindy to a big swing band, and thought everything was swell. Another twenty-year cycle gave us the Hippie with her bare feet, bell-bottomed jeans, and waist-length hair. She danced the Frug to acid rock and thought it was groovy to do her own thing.

Now, in the eighties, we have the Valley Girl. Fer shurr.

Originally, the term *Valley Girl* (and the male counterpart, *Valley Dude*) applied to teenagers from Southern California's San Fernando Valley, a pubescent paradise of sunshine, shopping malls, and freeways that all lead to the beach. The overprivileged adolescents of these Los Angeles suburbs managed to parlay a genius for spending money on cars, clothes, and amusements and a gift for linguistic mayhem into a lifestyle that has swept the nation from shopping mall to shopping mall. Today, no community is safe from the Valley cult, and no matter where you live in these United States you may find yourself harboring a Valley Girl or Dude under your very own roof.

A good way to determine whether or not you have a Val

in your house is to find out how often the suspected Val really *is* in the house. The natural habitat of both Valley Girls and Dudes is the shopping mall, invariably known in Val parlance as the Galleria. The Galleria environment encourages the Vals to exercise their gift for spending money. Clothes, food, arcade games, and various items of electronic paraphernalia are all fair game for the consumption-minded Val. Most Valley conversation, in fact, revolves around *things:* who has what, who's is better, who has more. Even members of the opposite sex are considered from this acquisitive perspective. A good-looking boyfriend ("buf babe" in Valspeak) can be displayed with as much proprietary pride as a new necklace.

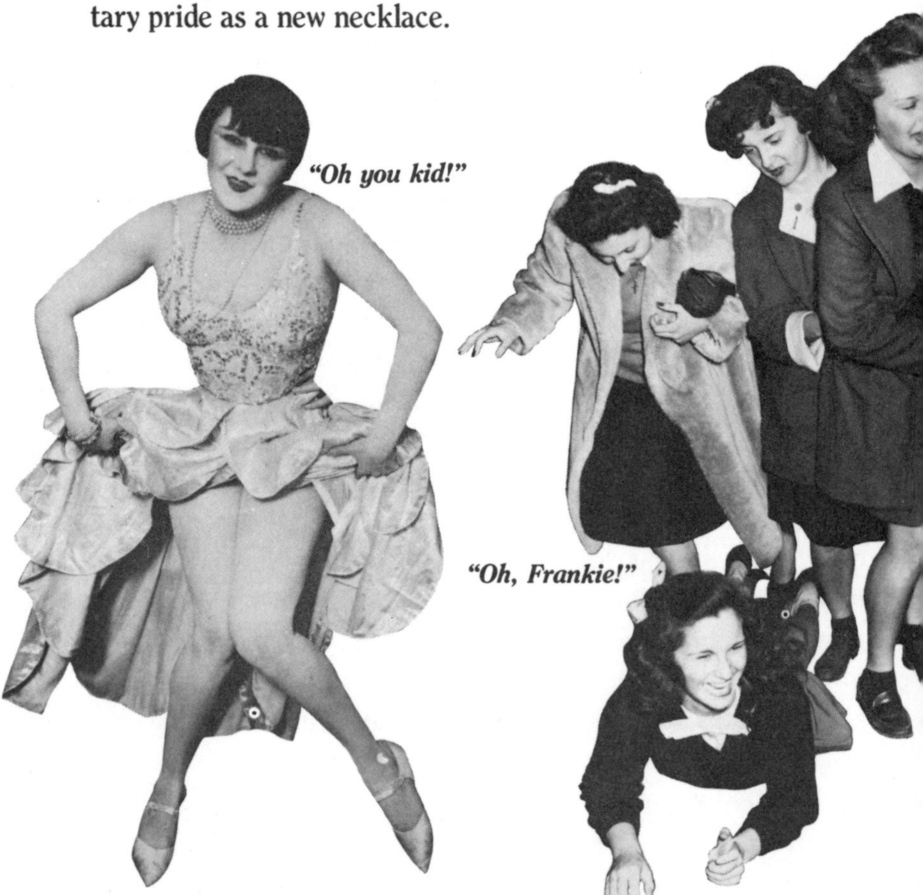

Ultimately, even the Val language is subject to a kind of verbal materialism, with words and phrases used not so much for their intrinsic meaning as for their indication of membership in the Val world. But more on this later. First let's examine the warning signs of Valleyism.

The transformation from a normal teenager to a full-blown fer-shurr Valley Girl does not occur overnight. Like the slow metamorphosis of a caterpillar into a butterfly—or a cold into galloping pneumonia—the emergence of a Valley Girl in your own home can take place under your nose without your noticing it until it's too late. How does it happen?

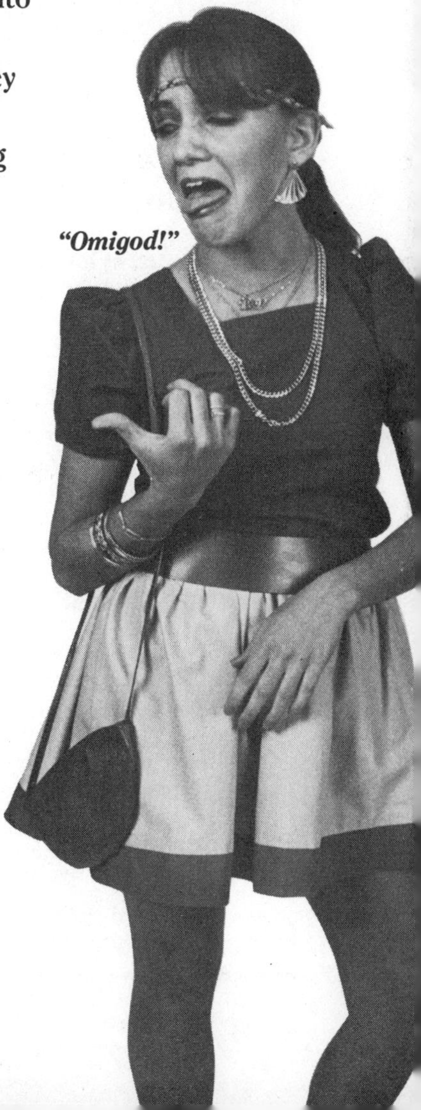

"Omigod!"

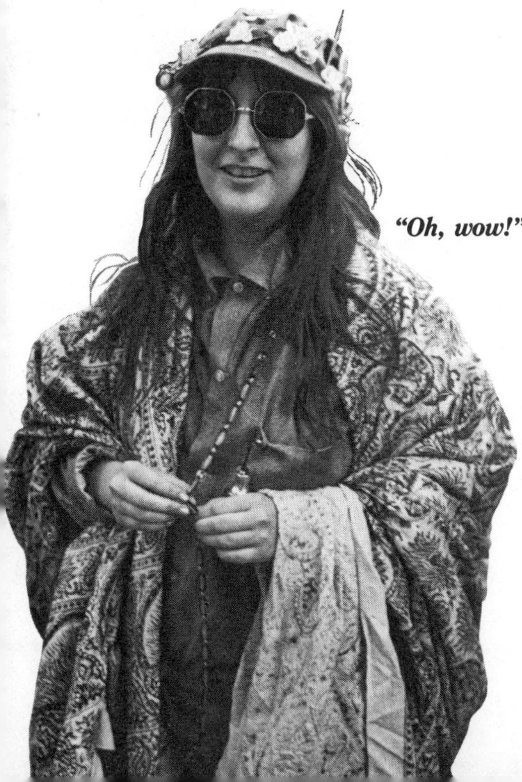

"Oh, wow!"

PRE-VAL PHASE

CLOTHING
The pre-Valley Girl's approach to dress is functional: tennis clothes for tennis, riding clothes for riding, swim suit for swimming. Her clothes are a means, not an end in themselves. For doing nothing in particular she likes an old pair of jeans and a simple top.

MAKEUP
She uses only the bare minimum (clear nail polish, a touch of lipstick), and only on special occasions. She does not consider a phone call a special occasion.

SPEECH
The pre-Val speaks American English. Her speech may have a touch of local color—a Southern drawl or a Texas twang—but she can be perfectly understood, even by people over sixteen who have never heard of Pat Benatar.

ATTITUDE
The pre-Val is helpful, cheerful, obedient, thrifty, courteous, and kind. In spirit she would make a perfect Girl Scout, but—an ominous warning sign—she can't stand those uniforms.

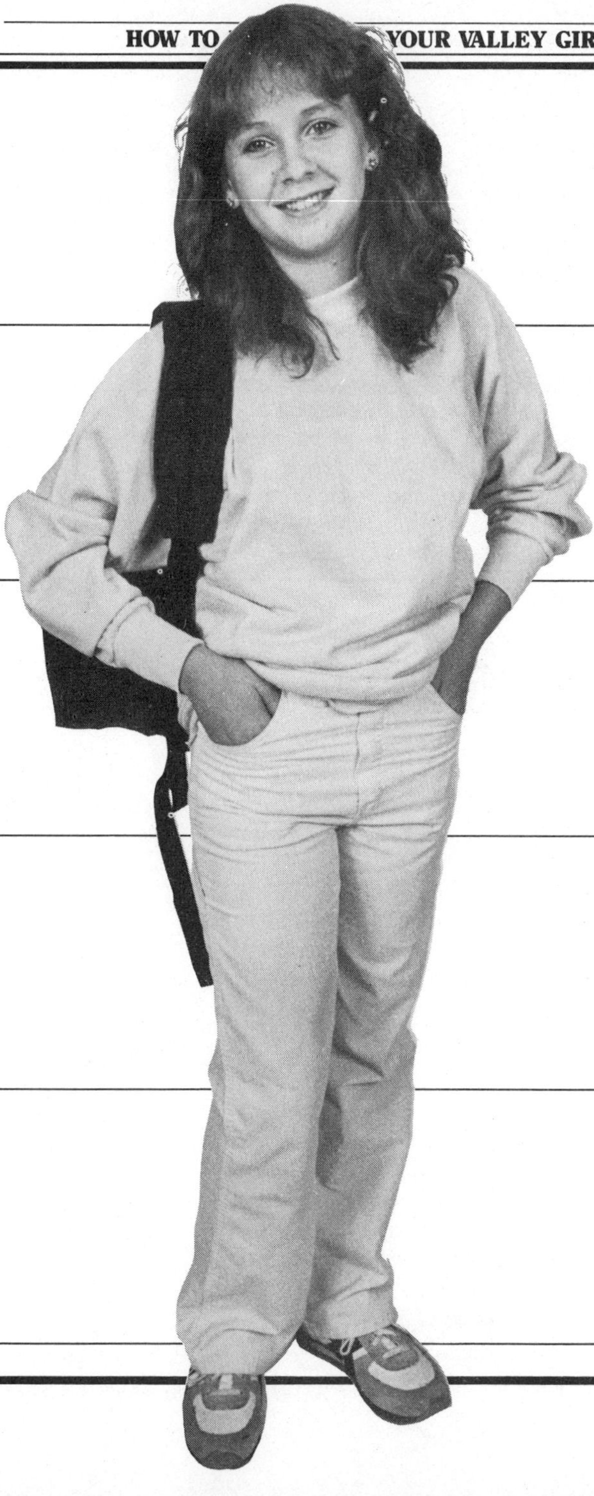

PHASE ONE

THE CALL TO COLORS

CLOTHING

In its earliest stage, the manifestations of the Valley style often seem harmless, even cute. The emerging Valley Girl begins to display a preoccupation with matching colors. Her color-coordinated miniskirt, top, and anklet socks may give parents an illusory sense that their daughter is developing good taste.

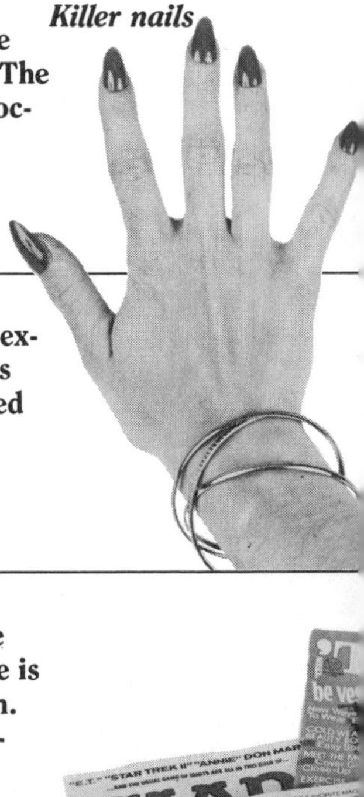

Killer nails

MAKEUP

The early Val passion for color coordination extends to cosmetics as well as clothes. Her lips and fingernails begin to display a shade of red as bright as a morning sunrise.

LANGUAGE

Speech, too, takes on dramatic colors. In the initial phase of the Val metamorphosis, there is a disarming tendency toward verbal inflation. Nothing is simply good or bad anymore; suddenly everything must be either *totally* awesome or *sooooo* gross.

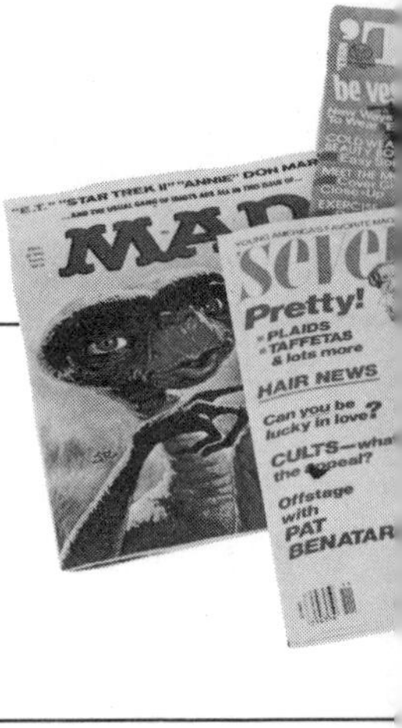

ATTITUDE

The Phase I Valley Girl is still a member of your family, speaking recognizable English. Caught at this stage, her transformation might still be nipped in the bud, although any too-vigorous attempt to do so is liable to result in a Punk or New Wave mutation, the deprogramming of which is beyond the scope of any book.

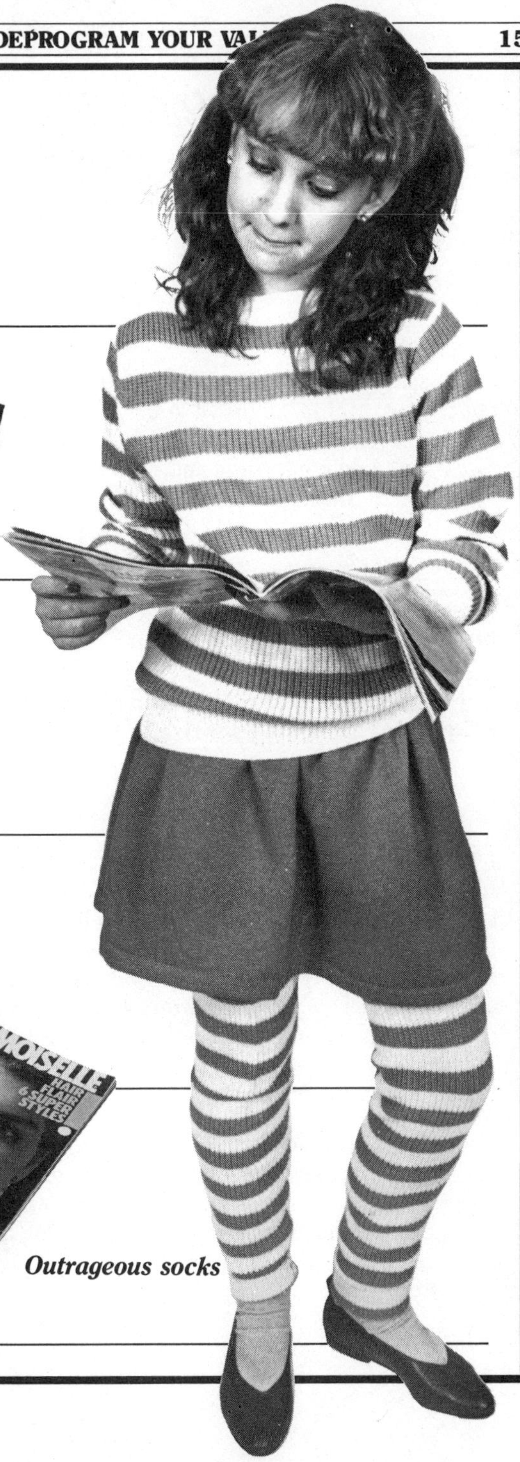

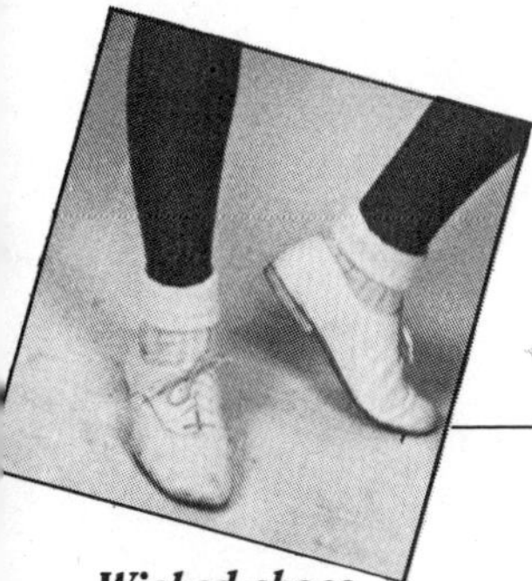

Wicked shoes

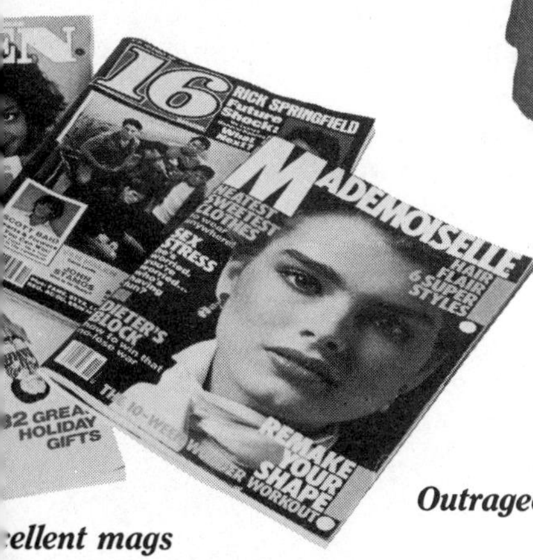

Outrageous socks

ellent mags

PHASE TWO

THE SHINING

CLOTHING

In the second phase of the Valley Girl metamorphosis, everything seems to get shiny. Pumps and purse glow with the sheen of patent leather. The flash of gold earrings and gold chains threatens to blind the onlooker.

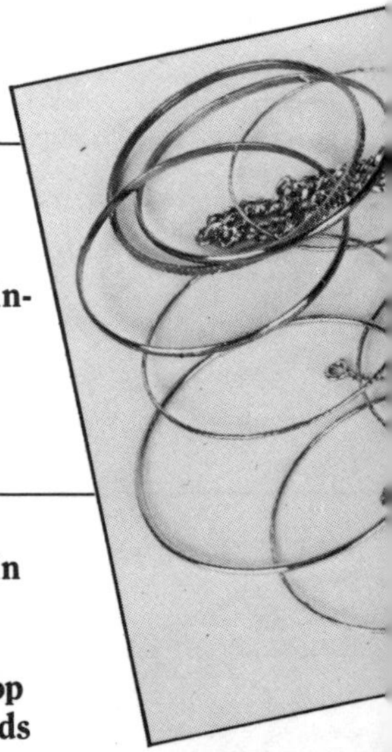

MAKEUP

The glossiness of the second phase is particularly apparent on the lips, which now appear bright enough to read by. Toenails as well as fingernails gleam with multiple layers of polish.

LANGUAGE

Although the words are still English, they begin to display some of the distortion of a body reflected in a funhouse mirror. Common expressions like "Oh my God!" and "for sure" develop dazzling roller-coaster rhythms, while the words surrounding them become submerged in a mumbled monotone.

ATTITUDE

There is an increased interest in boys, but a Val's most intense relationship is with her own reflection. If you ask an offspring at this stage whether she considers herself a Valley Girl, she will most likely respond, "No way!"
But she is.

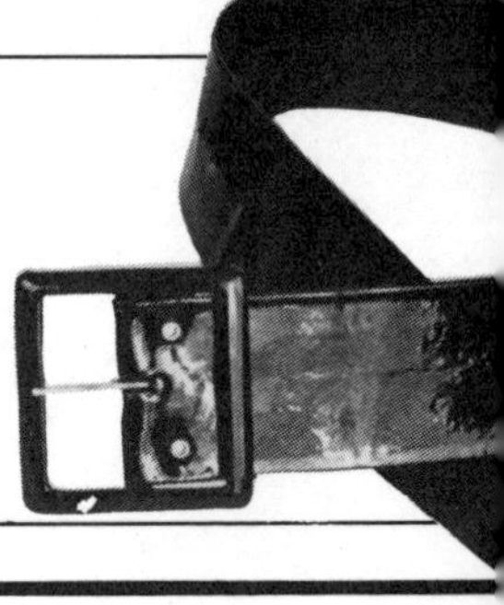

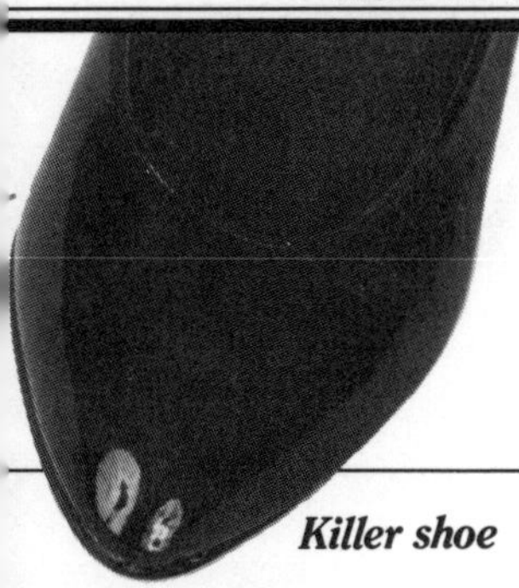

Killer shoe

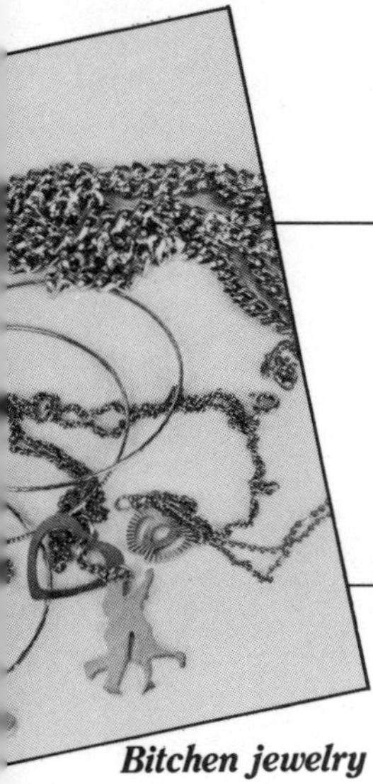

Bitchen jewelry

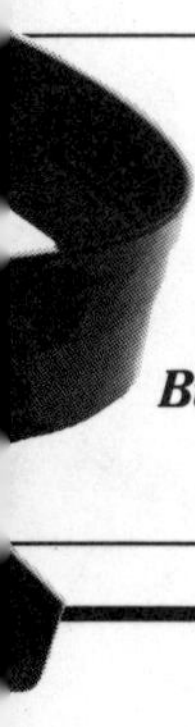

Buf belt

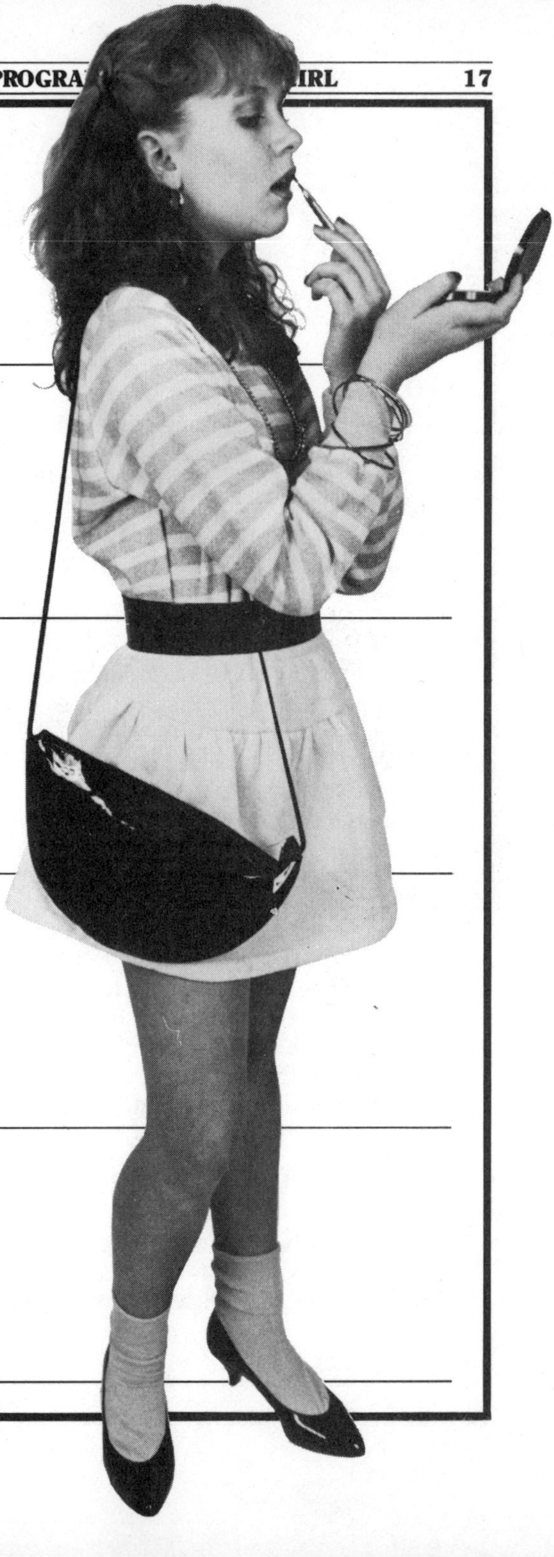

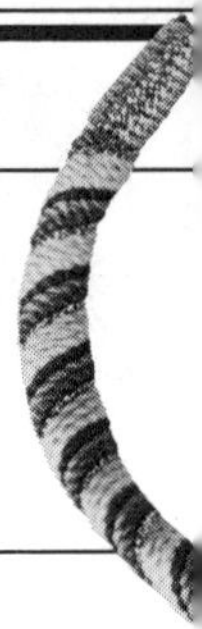

PHASE THREE

TIGHTENING UP

CLOTHING

This phase of the Valley transformation is marked by the phenomenon known as constriction. The gold chains multiply until their sheer weight threatens to choke the wearer; belts become thicker and tighter. And a headband hugs the Val skull, leading parents to worry about the possibility of brain damage.

MAKEUP

The constriction of the neck chains and headband appears to make the eyes bulge out, an effect heightened by the uninhibited application of shadow, liner, and mascara. The face, already tightened by the headband, seems even less elastic under layers of blusher, foundation, and powder.

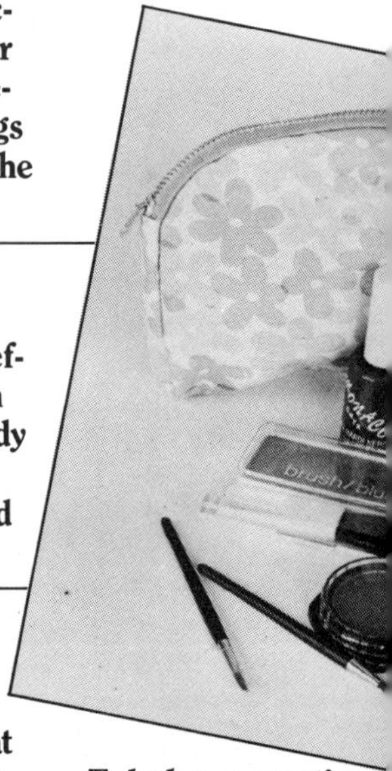

Tubular cosmetics

LANGUAGE

Speaking is now also constricted. The mouth hardly moves except to shift a wad of bubble gum from one side to the other. The words that do manage to emerge appear on the surface to be regulation English—"tubular," "radical," "shine"—but they no longer mean what the dictionary promises they should.

ATTITUDE

At this stage, the emerging Val is aggressively bored. She may also begin to develop the delusion that she lives in California, even if the Valley she actually inhabits is that of the Mississippi. You, too, may wish she lived in California.

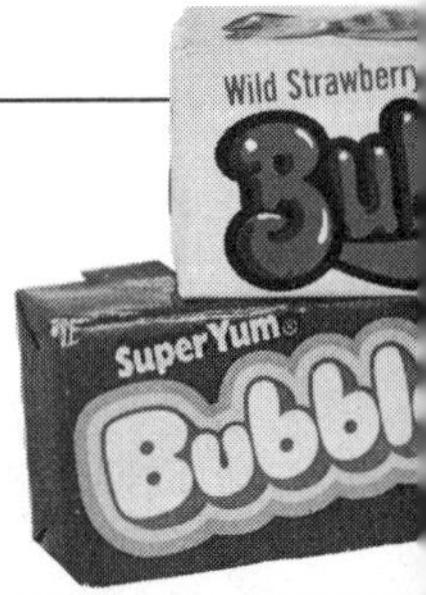

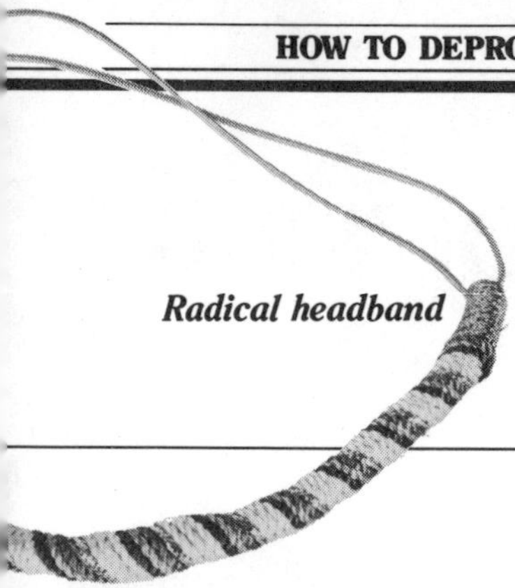

Radical headband

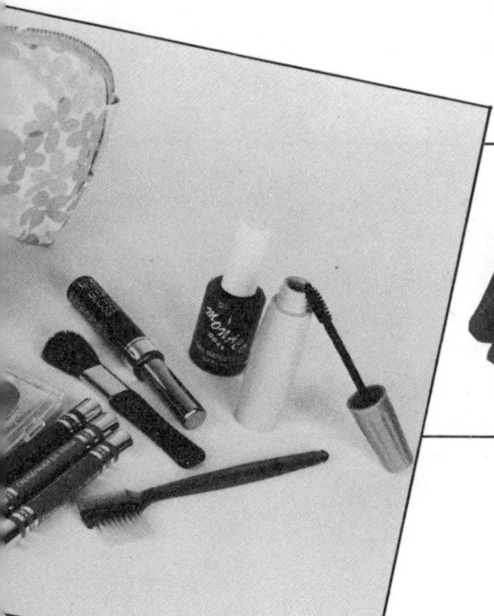

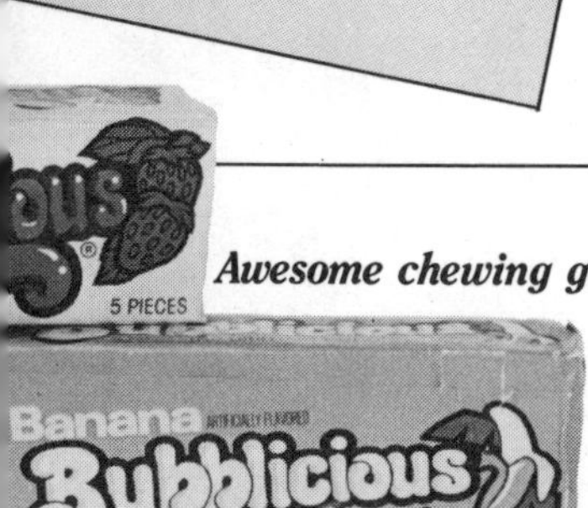

Awesome chewing gum

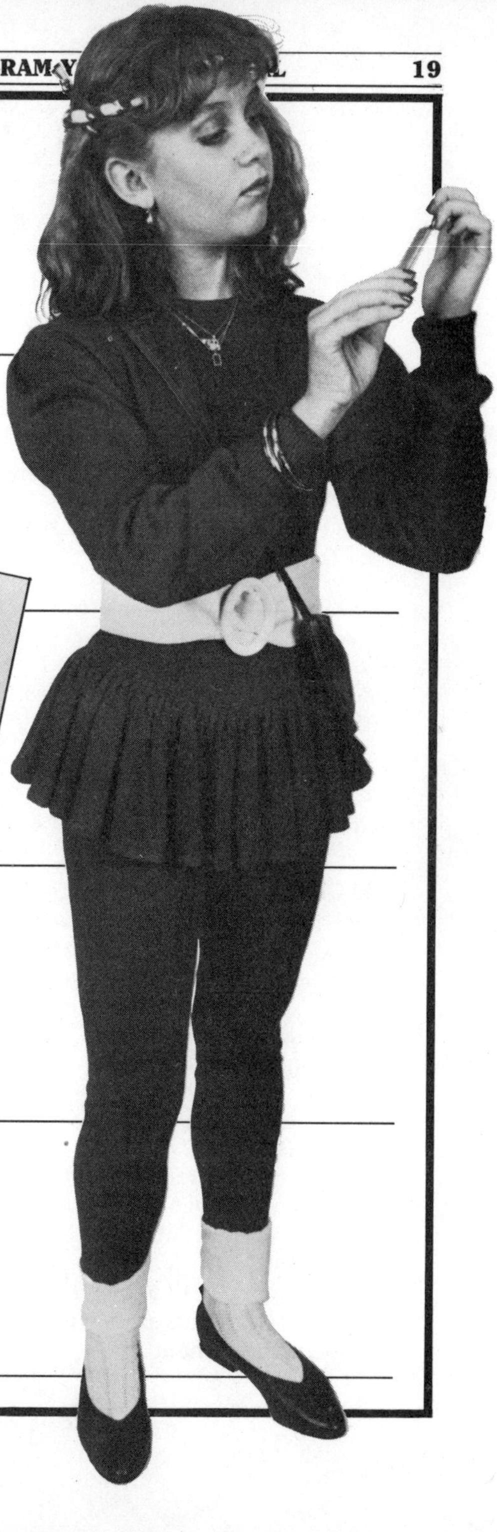

PHASE FOUR

THE SPROUTING

CLOTHING

In the final phase, things begin to sprout. Ruffles and frills blossom everywhere, like the petals of a tropical flower. Earrings seem to grow bigger, like leaves, and the eyes disappear behind reflecting wraparound sunglasses.

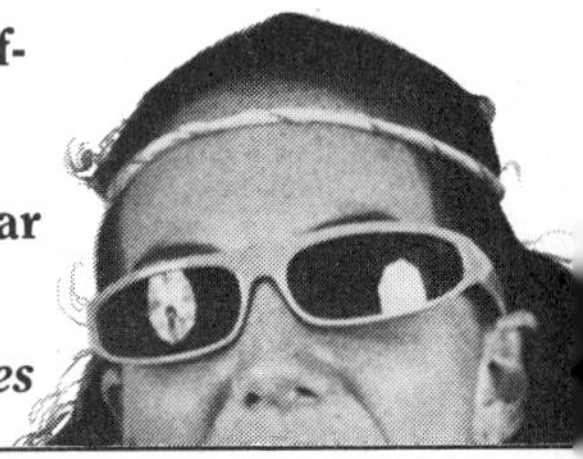

Insane shades

MAKEUP

Blush is now deep enough to ski through, and the sprouting motif expresses itself in the hair with the emergence of little tufts and bunches.

LANGUAGE

Speech at this stage appears to have entirely lost touch with English. It bursts with such unique coinages as "buf," "gnarley," and "grody." These are embedded in a rapid-fire fusillade of "likes" and "y'knows" as thick as a Val's makeup.

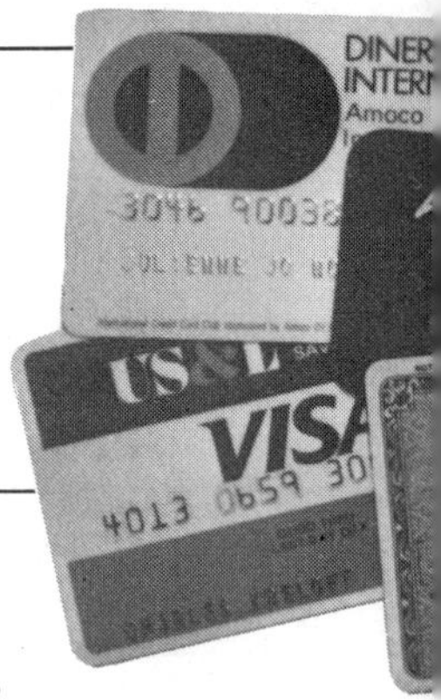

ATTITUDE

Parents and children have now become a complete embarrassment to one another. They are spared excessive contact by the fact that the full-blown Valley Girl spends at least as much time at the shopping mall as she does at home, and the charge-card bills are a small price to pay for not having her around.

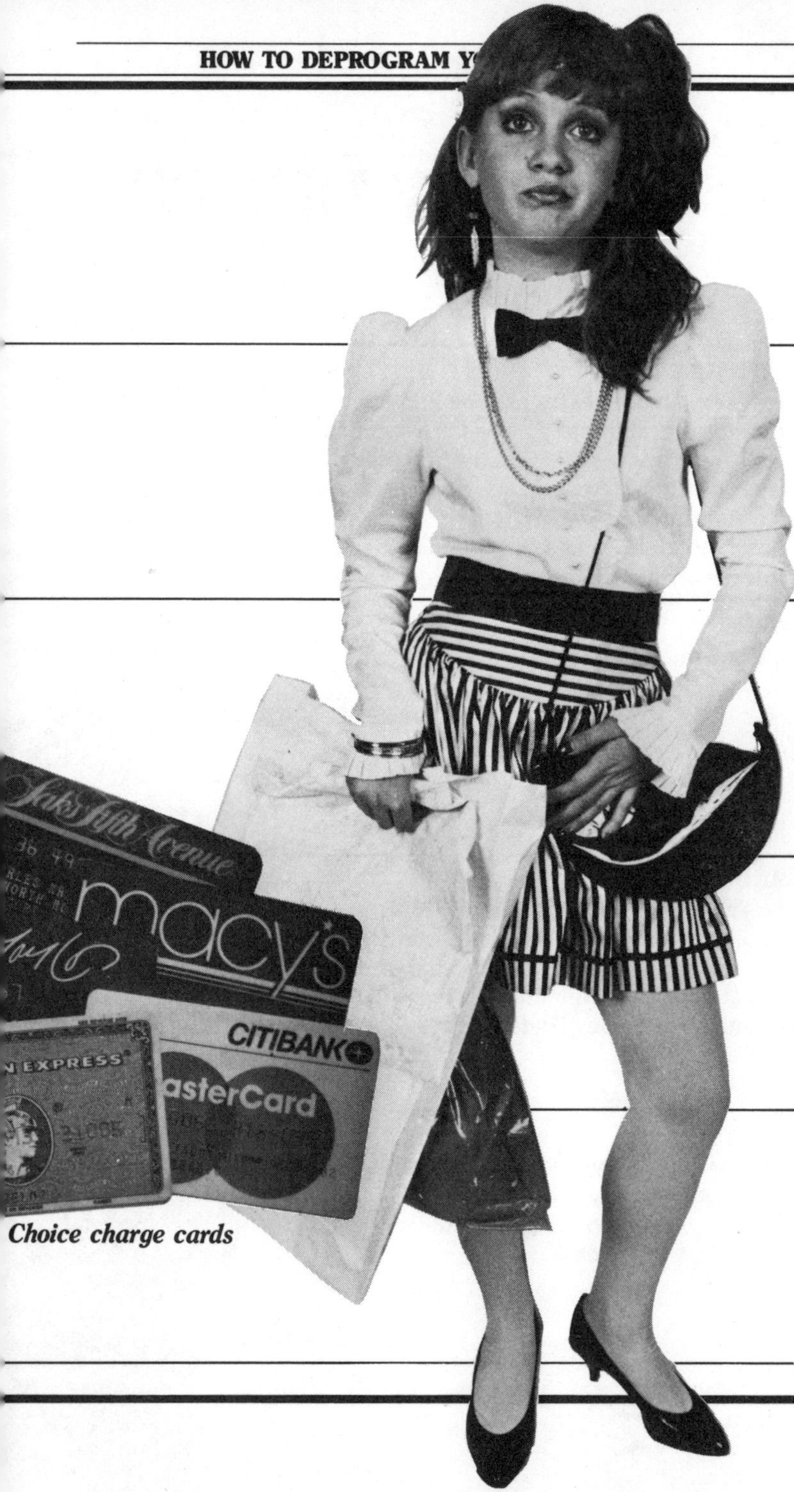

Choice charge cards

VALLEY DUDES

CLOTHING

The Valley Dude dresses as if he had just come from—or was about to go to—the beach. He wears sunglasses, sandals, a T-shirt (usually with rolled-up sleeves), jeans, and for formal occasions an oversized Hawaiian shirt. He sports a bandanna, either as a headband or tied around his jeans at the thigh—the tourniquet look.

MAKEUP

Sun screen.

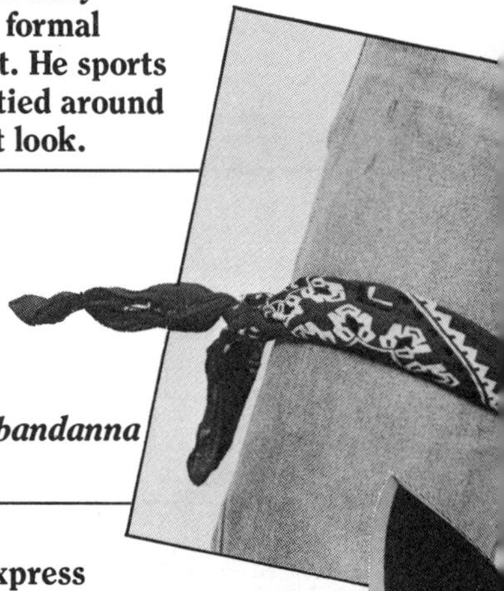

Bitchen bandanna

LANGUAGE

The Valley Dude finds it difficult to express himself in words, even Valspeak words. His monotone is more pronounced than that of his female counterpart, but since he says so little it is less annoying. Valley Dudes address each other as "Dude."

ATTITUDE

Like sharks, Valley Dudes need continual forward motion to keep their brains alive. Without wheels or surf propelling them onward, they lapse into a near coma.

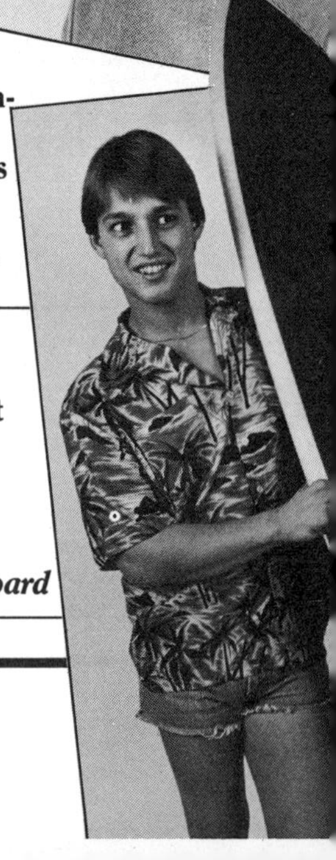

Buf board

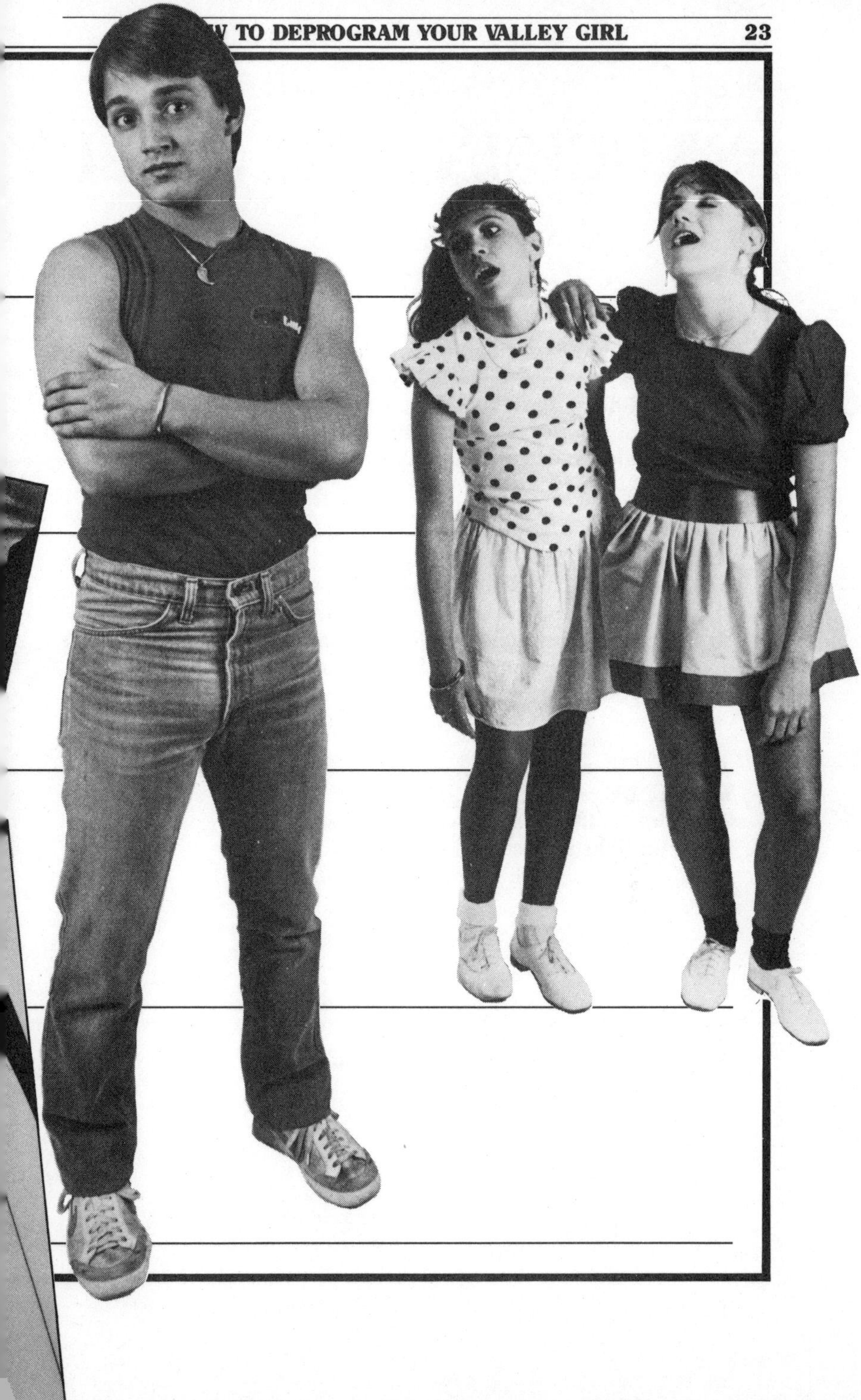

TERMINAL PHASE

STUCK IN THE VALLEY

CLOTHES

Whatever the vagaries of fashion, the Terminal Phase Valley Girl—now the Valley Matron—wears her mini and tights all the way into the twenty-first century. Only the mini isn't so mini and the tights keep getting tighter.

MAKEUP

The Terminal Phase Val tops off her collection of cosmetics with a few drums of industrial-strength skin conditioner. Instead of tans, she and her friends compare totally awesome face-lifts.

LANGUAGE

The words of the Valspeak vocabulary endure, but definitions shift subtly. A "way vicious babe" is any guy with his own teeth and hair.

ATTITUDE

She may be on her second husband and third child, but the world is still her high school. She just thinks of herself as being in the thirty-fifth grade.

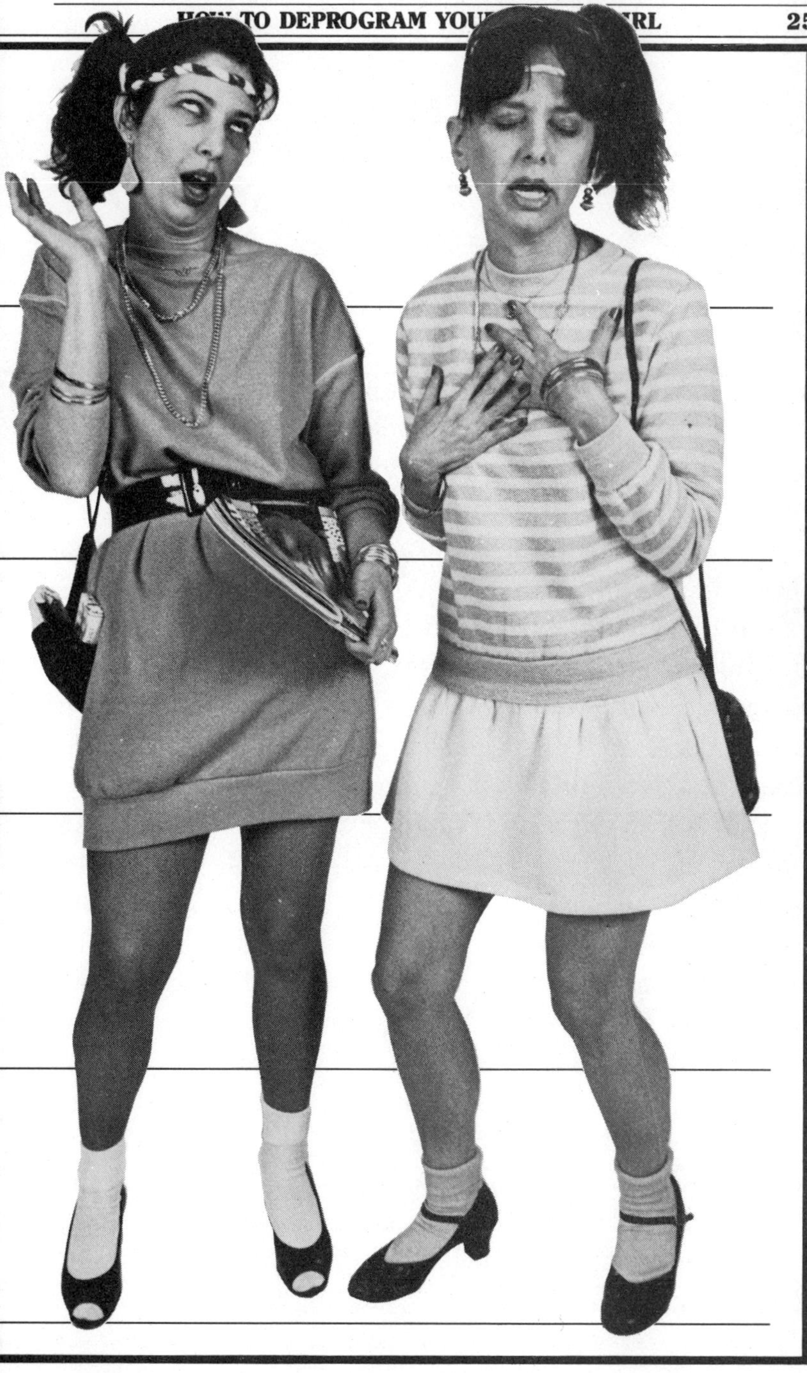

VALLEY VOCABULARY

Valley Girls and Dudes sometimes give the impression that they have started speaking a foreign language. Never mind that they may have never been farther from home than the nearest beach or shopping mall; somehow, they appear to have mastered a complex new idiom with its own vocabulary, syntax, and accent.

In reality, Valspeak is only a jargon, not a language. There are no more than a few dozen words in the Valspeak lexicon at any given moment that a native speaker of American English would not recognize. But, like doctor talk or lawyer talk, what you hear doesn't always mean what you think it does. And Valspeak carries an additional disadvantage. It is only useful for application to an extremely limited range of human experience—boys, cars, clothes, eating, and throwing up. This makes it more or less adequate for expressing delight at the physical appearance of an attractive young man driving by in a Corvette with a surfboard strapped to the back ("Wo! Like, buf Dude! Y'know, like, cruisemobile, huh?"); it is, however, less than appropriate when describing a presidential motorcade or a NASA astronaut ("Wo! Like, buf Dude! Y'know, like, cruisemobile, huh?"). And a discourse on aerodynamics, economic recovery, or jurisprudence in Valspeak (although few Valspeakers would engage in such a dialogue) would be confined to the broadest expressions of approval or disapproval ("Writ of habeas corpus? Like, gross me *out*!")

VALLEY VERBS

What do Vals do when they're not talking on the telephone? Not much. Below is a list of words describing typical Val activities.

bail: to leave

barf: to throw up

pig out: to overeat

rolf: to throw up

scarf out: to overeat

shine: to leave

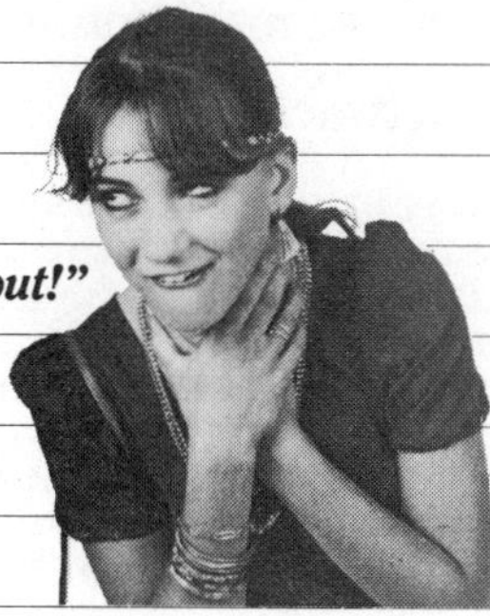

"Barf me out!"

INANIMATE OBJECTS

Valley life is built around *things.* Some of the most important are:

billies: money; from *dollar bills*

boogie board: a short surfboard

cruisemobile: a desirable car

Galleria: a shopping mall

Heinies: Heineken beer

keggers: kegs of beer (any brand)

Lowies: Lowenbrau beer

mini: a short skirt

UV's: the sun's rays; from *ultraviolet*

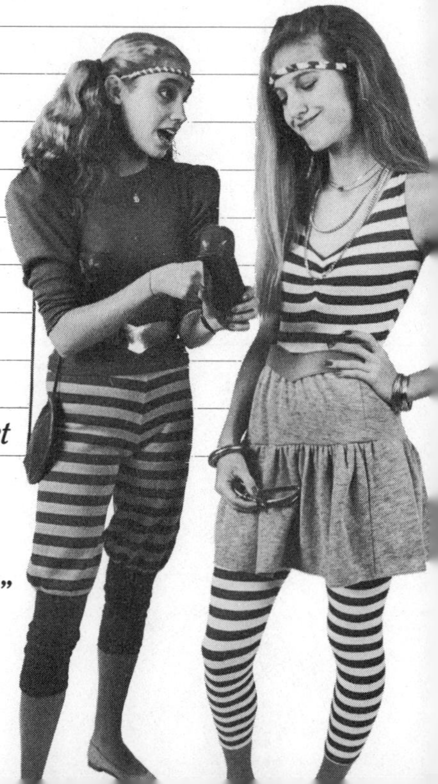

"I got the billies!"

ANIMATE OBJECTS

Almost as important as things are people, whom Vals regard with the same acquisitiveness as they do clothes or cars. Some of the merchandise:

babe: attractive member of either sex

beastie: unattractive member of the female sex

bufu: homosexual, regardless of looks

fox: attractive member of either sex

geek: unattractive member of either sex

goober: unintelligent member of the male sex

Melvin: unattractive member of the male sex

nurd: unattractive member of the male sex

Poindexter: intelligent, but unattractive, member of the male sex

zod: unattractive member of the male sex

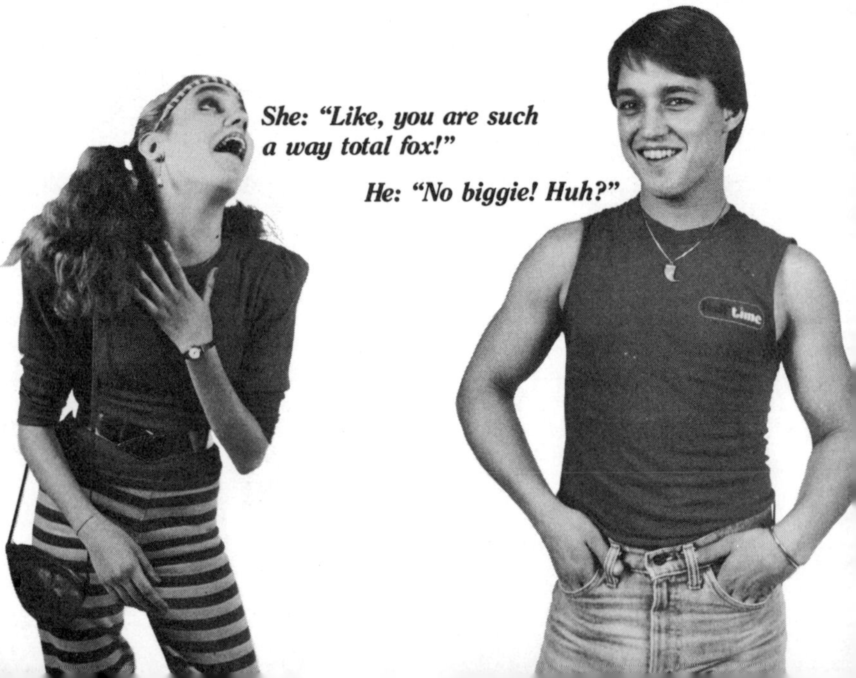
She: "Like, you are such a way total fox!"
He: "No biggie! Huh?"

WORDS OF APPROVAL OR DISAPPROVAL

Valspeak is a language of black and white. Fine distinctions and shades of gray have no place here. The either/ors:

awesome: good

beige: boring

bitchen: good

buf: good-looking

choice: good

excellent: good

gnarley: disgusting

grody: disgusting

gross: disgusting

insane: good

killer: good

outrageous: good

radical (or **rad**)**:** good

skanky: disgusting

tubular: good

vicious: good-looking

wicked: good

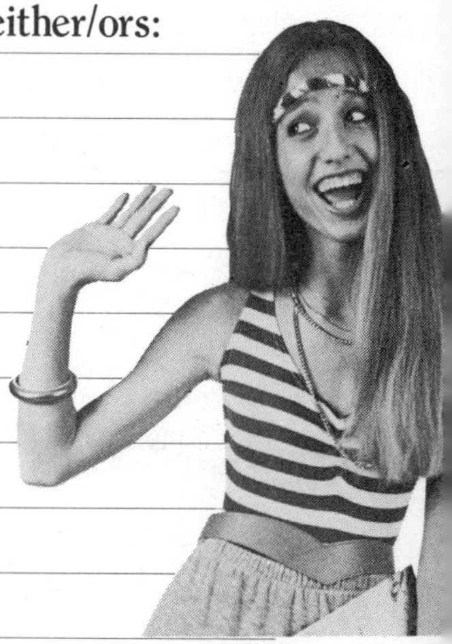

"Radical!"

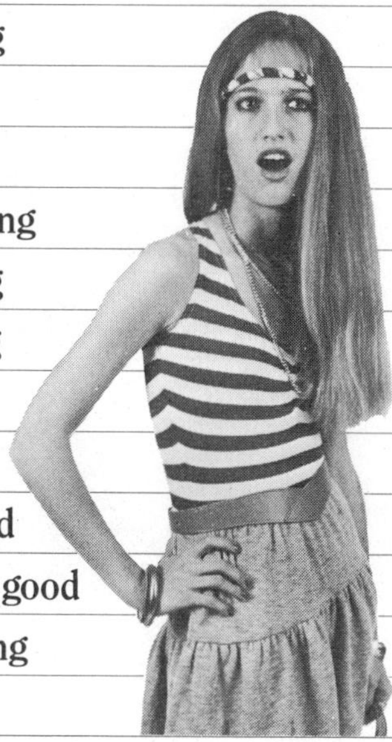

"Awesome!"

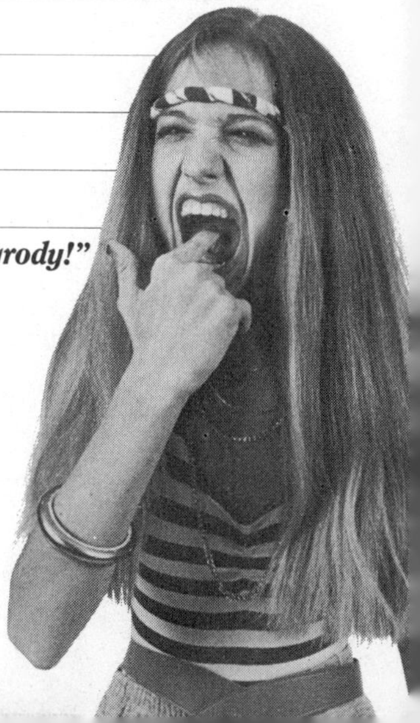

"Ew, grody!"

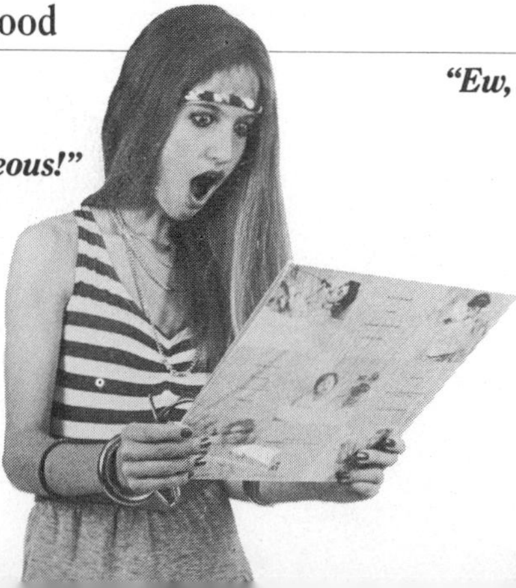

"Outrageous!"

STATES OF MIND

Normal waking consciousness is held in low regard in the Val world, and practically any deviation from that *beige* state is highly esteemed. Some standard aberrations:

amped: up

freaked out: crazed

hyper: up

jazzed: up

juiced: drunk

psyched: up

stoked: up

thrashed: down

tweeked: drunk

wasted: drunk

zeeked: crazed

zooned out: crazed

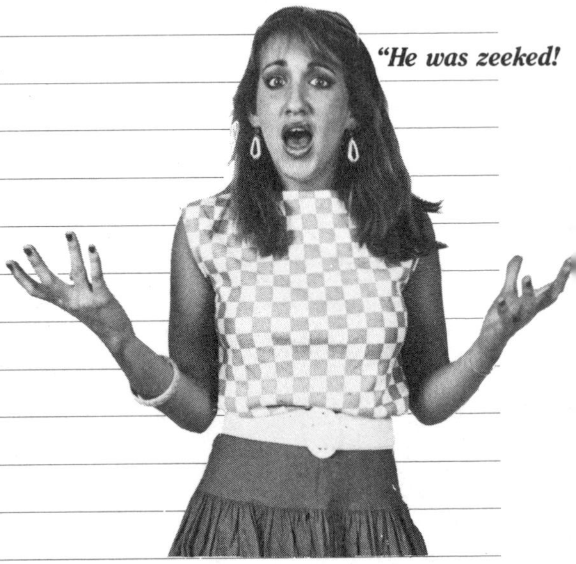

"He was zeeked!

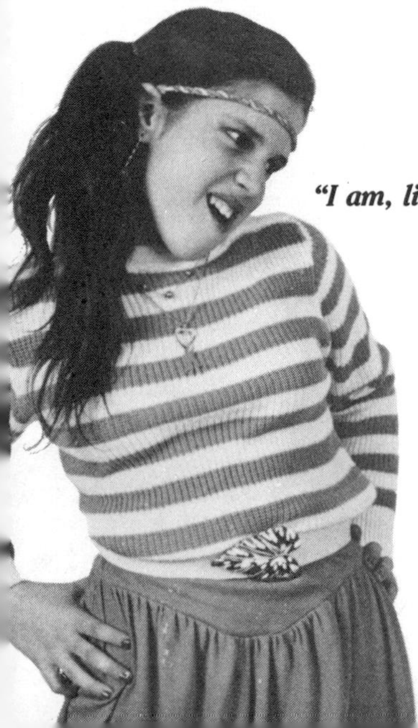

"I am, like, sooooo freaked out! Huh?"

EXCLAMATORY PHRASES

The intensity of Valley life requires frequent expressions of agreement, disagreement, and nausea. Some ready-made epithets:

bag your face! You're so ugly that I'm nauseated

barf me out: I'm nauseated

ew! I'm nauseated

fer shurr: I agree

gag me with a spoon: I'm nauseated

I'm (so) sure: I disagree

no way: I disagree

omigod! I'm surprised (and possibly nauseated as well)

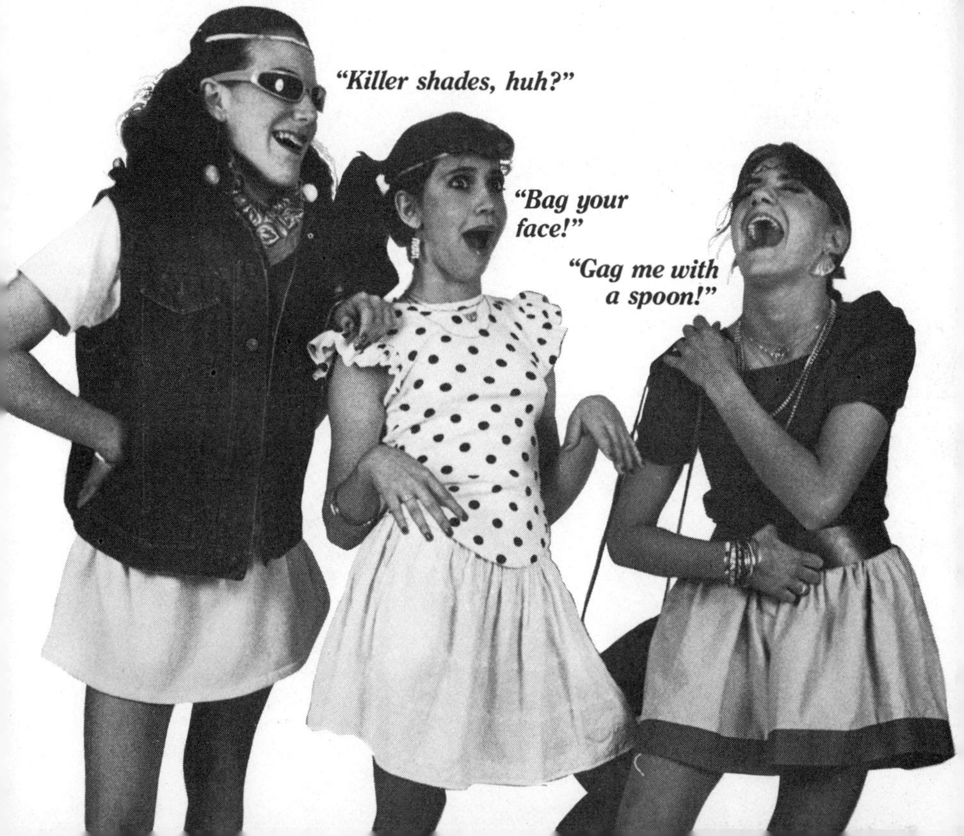
"Killer shades, huh?"
"Bag your face!"
"Gag me with a spoon!"

HELPER WORDS

These words are the lip gloss of Valspeak. They are used to highlight what otherwise might be mistaken for relatively trivial observations. Helper words are generally strung together into gaudy chains; they are rarely used by themselves. To describe a babe as "totally buf" is to damn him with faint praise. Unless he's really a mega-geek, proper Valspeak etiquette calls for at least a double helping ("way totally buf") or, better yet, a quadruple ("really sooooo way totally buf") to do him justice.

Helper words are the most strongly inflected words in Valspeak; in fact, they are probably the *only* inflected words. All of them mean "very."

completely

fully

mega

major

maximum (to the max)

mondo

really

sooooo

totally

way

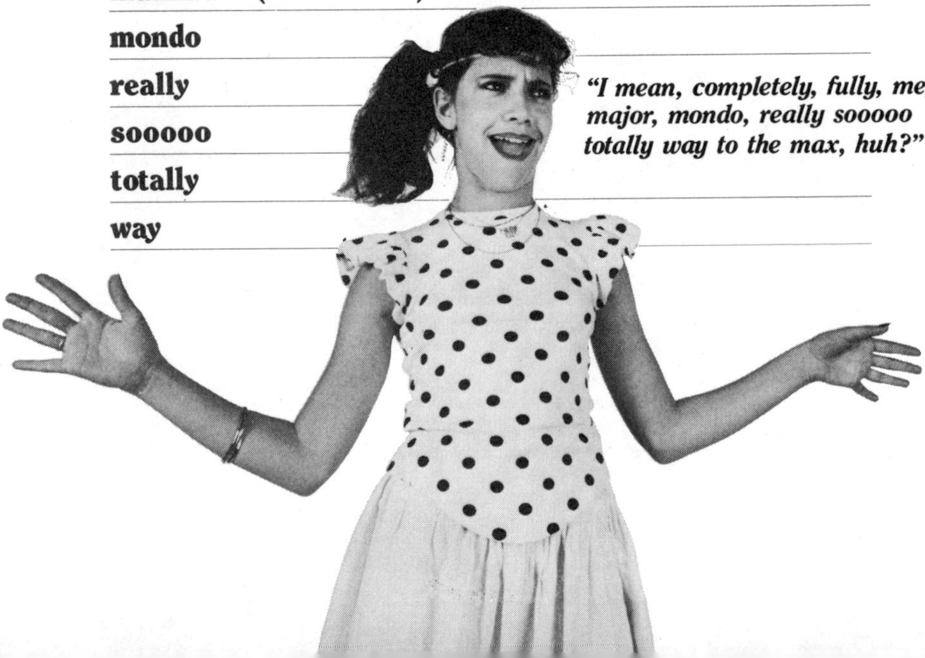

"I mean, completely, fully, meg major, mondo, really sooooo totally way to the max, huh?"

FILLER WORDS

These words and sounds are hardly exclusive to Valspeak, but they play a major part in practically any Valley utterance. They account for what communications scientists would call the grotesquely low signal-to-noise ratio in Valspeak—the words that you can actually hear are the least important in the sentence. Like helper words, they can be strung together like beads on a chain. In fact, *entire* Valley sentences can be formed using only filler words (e.g., "O.K., huh, like, y'know, like I dunno, y'know?")

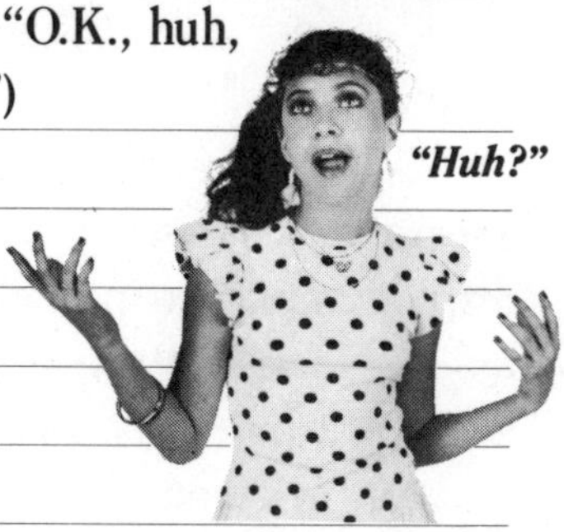

"Huh?"

huh

I dunno

I mean

like

O.K.

so (not to be confused with the helper word *sooooo*)

y'know

MAKING VALSPEAK SENTENCES

Valspeak has a syntax all its own, or, more properly, none. To make Valspeak sentences, you need not pay attention to such grammatical niceties as subjects, predicates, and objects. Valspeak sentences are constructed by jamming together as many of the above words as will fit on a breath. A typical, all-purpose deep stucture for such a sentence might be:
[filler]—[exclamation]—[filler]—[filler]—[helper]—[helper]—[approval or disapproval word]—[animate object]—[filler].

This structure will generate such Valspeak sentences as: "Like, Omigod! I mean like way totally wicked dude, y'know!" or: "I mean, barf me out! Y'know, like really mega-geek, huh?"

VALSPEAK ANATOMY

The assorted sounds known collectively as Valspeak are produced by a mechanism remarkably similar to that which produces human speech. To understand it, we can think of our Valley Girl as a long tube filled with air—literally tubular.

At the lower end of this teenaged tube is the respiratory apparatus, consisting of the diaphragm and the lungs. The diaphragm is a strip of elastic tissue, something like a really buf headband. When it contracts, it pulls the lungs down, allowing whatever happens to be in the atmosphere at the moment to come rushing into the pulmonary cavity. When the diaphragm relaxes it returns to its original position, expelling the contents of the lungs. This is known as breathing. It is an automatic reflex, like brushing the hair.

For Valley Girls, it seems, this simple process of inhaling oxygen and exhaling carbon dioxide is fraught with as many difficulties as trigonometry. This is not because Valley Girls lack coordination. They have no difficulty walking and chewing gum simultaneously, for example (though some may have difficulty walking without chewing gum).

In normal human speech, the speaker inhales, then talks on the exhalation, the words being carried on the stream of air emerging from the mouth like surfers riding the waves at Malibu. Valley speakers, by contrast, tend to inhale quickly and exhale all the air out of their lungs as rapidly as possible. *Then* they talk. This perverse procedure accounts for the characteristic last-gasp sound of some Valley speech.

Vals talk, it appears, not only *about* nothing, but *on* nothing. Speaking after exhalation compels Valspeakers to deliver their words at a pace that even a professional auctioneer would find hard to sustain.

VALLEY VOICE BOX

Up the tube from the lungs is the larynx, or voice box. On Valley Dudes this structure can be readily located as the Adam's apple. On Valley Girls it can be found just behind the gold necklace. Like the speaker of a mondo bitchen stereo system, the larynx is a vibrating membrane that determines the pitch, loudness, and tonal qualities of speech. It accounts for melody and color, the music behind the words.

In the media, Valspeak is often portrayed as being highly inflected, more sung than said. A simple *pull-eeeeeeze* delivered by an actress playing the stage version of a Valley Girl consists of a multi-octave arpeggio that could choke a Wagnerian diva. But, as most parents know, the true sound of Valspeak is more often a monotone that any self-respecting computer would be ashamed to produce. The words may be "totally awesome," but the music, as provided by the Val larynx, says only "pretty good." Vals think this sounds blasé and cool. Others hear dead fish.

NOSE AND MOUTH

At the top of the human tube is the articulatory mechanism—the mouth and its environs. This area contains the structures responsible for transforming raw voice into intelligible speech. What goes on here determines whether a vibrating column of air will emerge to the waiting world as "Omigod," "Bag your face," or "Barf me out!"

VALSPEAK VALVES

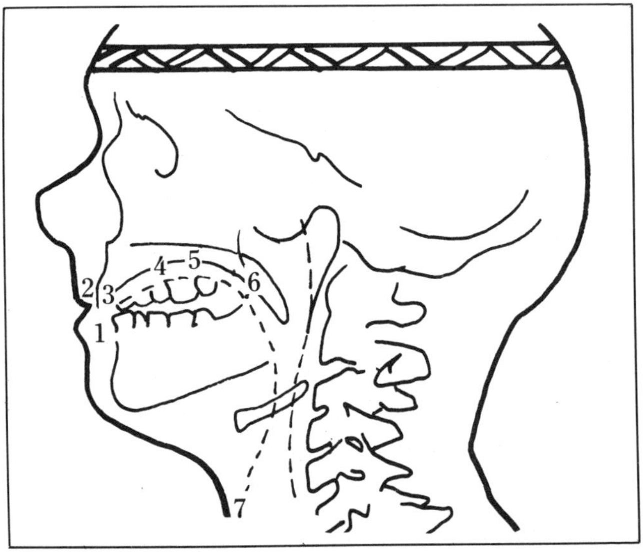

The sounds of Valspeak are formed in seven locations in the Val head, called musculoskeletal valves. The headband is silent.

1. Bilabial—*p,b,m*—preppie, babe, max
2. Labiodental—*f,v*—fer shurr, Val
3. Linguadental—*th*—thrashed
4. Lingua-alveolar—*t,d,n,l,s,z*—totally, Dude, nurd, like, sooooo, zod
5. Linguapalatal—*ch,j,sh,zh,r*—bitchen, jazzed, shine, rad
6. Linguavelar—*k,g,ng*—killer, grody, freaking
7. Glottal—*h* and vowel sound—Heinies

VALPRINTS

English meets Valspeak. All-time favorite Valley expressions "fer shurr," "toe-dully," and "omigod" *(top to bottom)* pose for spectrographic analysis. The normal pronounciation is on the left, Valspeak version on the right. Gnarley, huh?

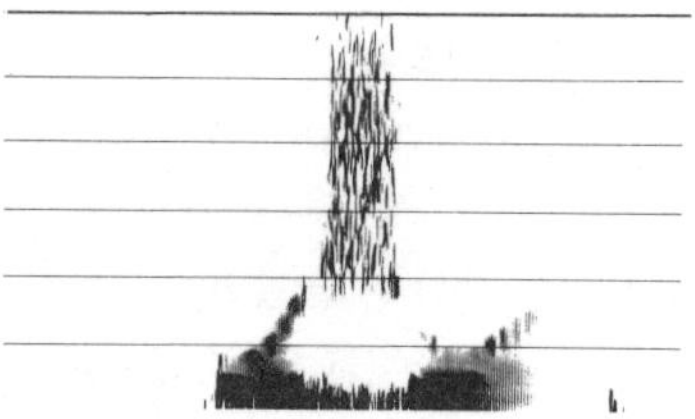

For sure

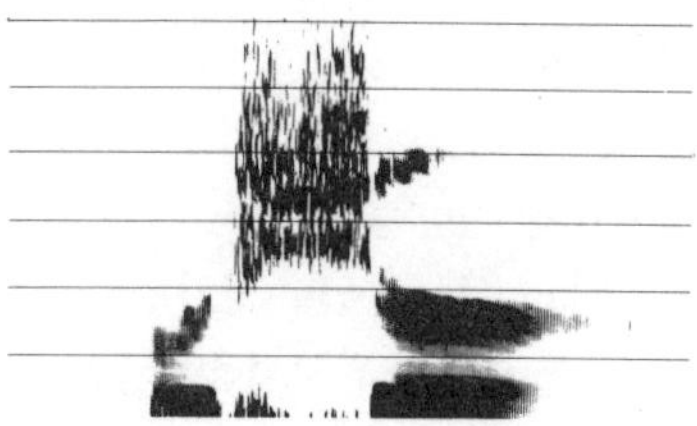

Fer shurr

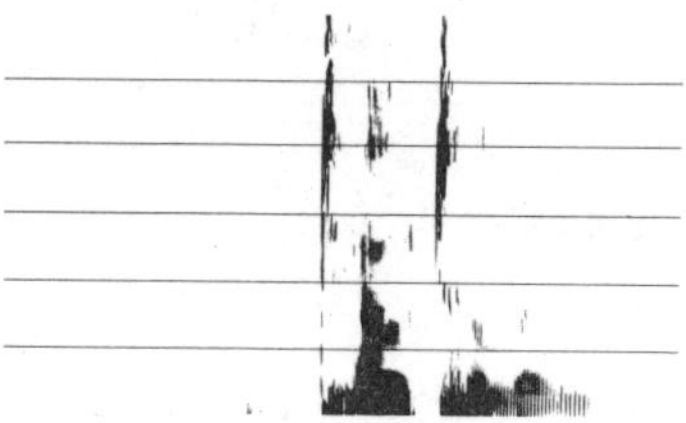

Totally

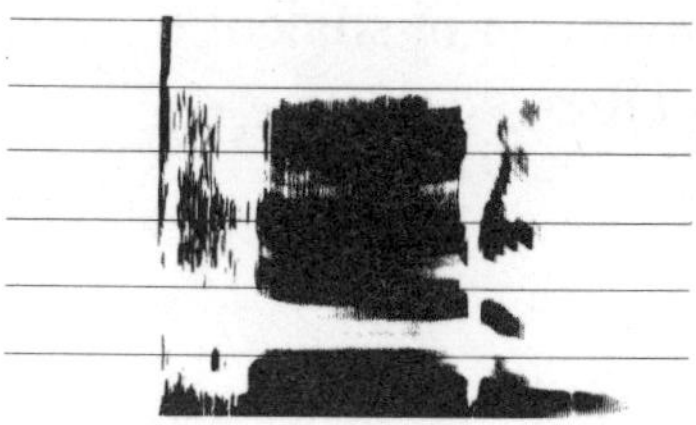

Toe-dully

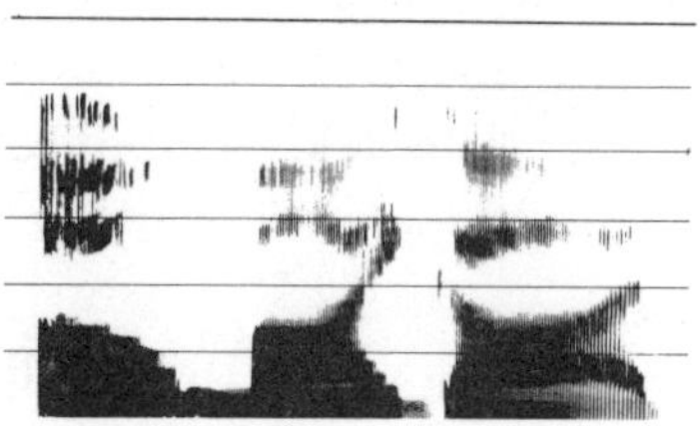

Oh my god

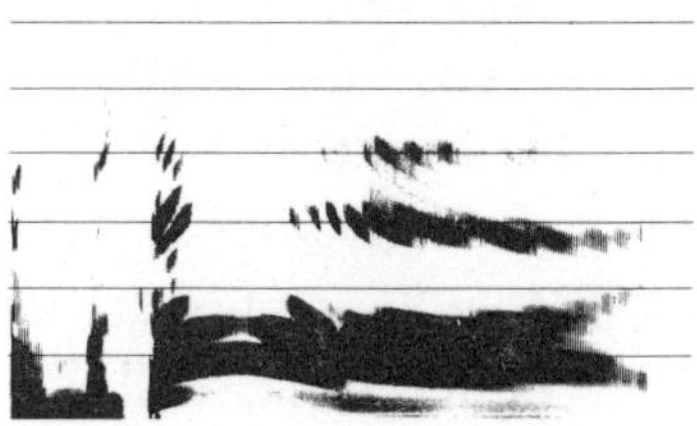

Omigod

Among the structures that come into play in forming words are the lips, the tongue, the teeth, the hard and soft palates, and the chewing gum.

Linguists have gone to a great deal of trouble to categorize the various vowel and consonant sounds that make up articulate speech [see page 36], but most of their efforts seem to have been wasted when it comes to Valspeakers, many of whom manage to swallow everything but their gum. Articulation is further thwarted by the Valspeaker's propensity for minimal mouth movements (any vigorous activity in that region might smear the lip gloss). As a result, parents find themselves saying "what?" almost as often as their offspring say "like."

And since the Valley mouth moves little and opens less, the sounds that Valspeakers produce have to find an alternate route to the atmosphere. This is usually the nose, with the result that a gathering of Valley Girls often sounds like a convention of student telephone operators or a flock of very well-dressed geese.

THE EARS

Although not generally thought of as organs of speech, the ears are an integral part of the human communication system; and they seem to be peculiarly defective in many Valspeakers. Like portable cassette players, Valspeakers seem able to put out sound but unable to take it in. They listen to one another reluctantly, and apparently only as a prelude to talking about themselves.

If Deborah says, "Like, y'know I just got this really bitchen lip gloss," the reply from Michelle will not be to ask where it came from, but instead to counter with "Fer shurr, like *my* lip gloss is really *sooooo* outrageous."

Val etiquette holds it particularly poor form to inquire about, or even register, the emotions of others.

Deborah: "My dad got hit by a car yesterday."

Michelle: "Ew, grody! Like what kind?"

THE FACE

Like the ears, the face plays an important role in speech, providing a visual display of the emotions and ideas being expressed. But most Valley Girls think of their faces as places to apply makeup. The idea of using them to convey any emotion other than nausea grosses them out to the max, and they prefer to look as expressionless as their utterances.

DE-PROGRAMMING

You've seen movies or news reports showing the techniques deprogrammers use to return terminally blissed-out cult zombies to the bosom of the family. The young victim may be kidnapped, isolated, starved, physically and psychologically assaulted. And as a Val parent, you may have fantasized that similar brute force might dissuade your teenager from her Valley ways. Have any of these tactics ever crossed your tormented mind?

- Lock her in her room and cut the cord of her Princess phone.
- Melt her credit cards.
- Soak her in nail polish remover and cold cream.
- Send her to a convent specializing in vows of silence and poverty.
- Exile her to an underdeveloped nation to learn frugality and an entirely new language.

Happily, such drastic measures are not necessary. The fact is that sooner or later, most Valley Girls and Dudes will want to change of their own accord. What seemed immensely appealing to a thirteen-year-old will not necessarily be so attractive at sixteen or seventeen. By that age most teenagers are coming to realize that there's a big world out there beyond the shopping mall and that they are going to have to find a place for themselves in it. Whether this means going to college or setting out on a career with rosier prospects than baby-sitting or grilling burgers to go, eventually the limitations of Valhood will become apparent to even the *totally* committed.

The catch is that just because they may eventually *want* to change doesn't mean that they'll be able to change. Hair and clothing styles, of course, can be easily altered. The orthodontist may at last pronounce their teeth straight and liberate them from their braces. Skin eruptions may clear up without major medical intervention. But speech patterns (and the habits of communication that go along with them) are not so easily outgrown. When you consider that many foreign-born Americans still bear their native accents despite years spent in this country developing language skills, you can appreciate the impossibility of slipping in and out of speech patterns in the same way you don each new season's fashions.

Still, the habits of Valspeak *can* be overcome with time and patience. Nagging is not the answer. A pat on the back is only a few vertebrae away from a kick in the butt, and far more effective.

The secret of deprogramming Valspeak or any other kind of speak is to become conscious of how—and why— you create the sounds and signs you use to communicate. As a parent, you can make the following exercises more effective by encouraging your Val to do them, and by participating in them yourself. Recording and playing back your voice may give you a few surprises about your own speech and communication patterns. Your jargon may not be as dense or distant as Valspeak, but the odds are you'll find yourself using expressions and phrases every bit as hard to understand. By working on your own speech habits, you'll be setting a good example for your Val while learning to communicate more effectively with her.

BREATHING: BACK TO BASICS

All speech depends on breathing, and every living person had better be able to breathe. But not all breathing is the same. Much of our respiratory behavior is learned, and learned badly. Dogs, cats, and babies all instinctively breathe using their abdomens. But as we get older and begin paying attention to teachers and parents who tell us to throw back our shoulders and stick out our chests, our breathing often becomes tighter, moving from the belly to the chest. This is called *clavicular breathing* and is neither as powerful nor efficient as the abdominal variety. Clavicular breathing provides pitifully little support for the voice, and professional singers—from Luciano Pavarotti to the Go-Go's—all have to learn (or relearn) to breathe using their abdominal muscles.

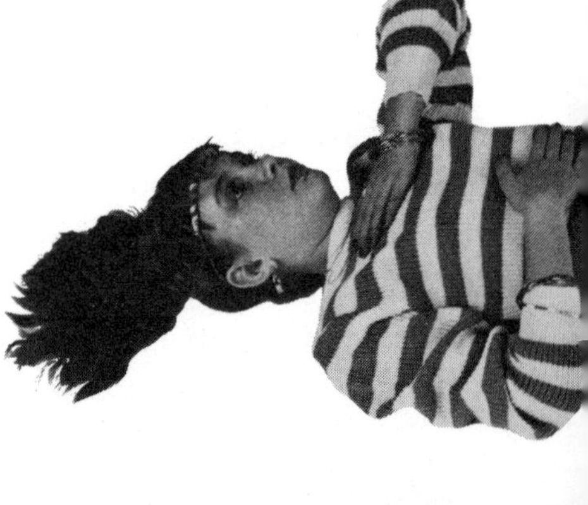

EXERCISE 1
TUMMY TEST

You can learn to breathe from your abdomen by lying on your back on a flat, comfortable surface like a firm bed, a carpeted floor, or even a nice sandy beach. Make sure your clothing is loose. Before beginning, try to become aware of your body and to relax those muscles that are tight. The chest and neck areas can be reservoirs of tension.

1. Once you're comfortable, place a hand, palm down, on your abdomen. To find the right place, sniff in three or four times, as if you had a runny nose. The spot on your belly that bounces when you do this is where your hand belongs. Place the palm of your other hand on your breastbone.

2. Take a breath through your nose for a slow count of five. Breathe evenly, letting the air flow in and feeling your tummy rise as your lungs fill up.

3. Hold the air in for another count of five, then let it out through your mouth, slowly and evenly, for a count of ten. All of this should be done as smoothly and comfortably as possible, without any sharp movements and without strain. Pay attention to the rising and falling of your abdomen. Try to breathe so that the only movement is under your abdominal hand; the hand on your upper chest should be completely still. The other muscles of your body should remain totally relaxed. Most people find this technique very soothing.

4. Repeat this exercise 20 times.

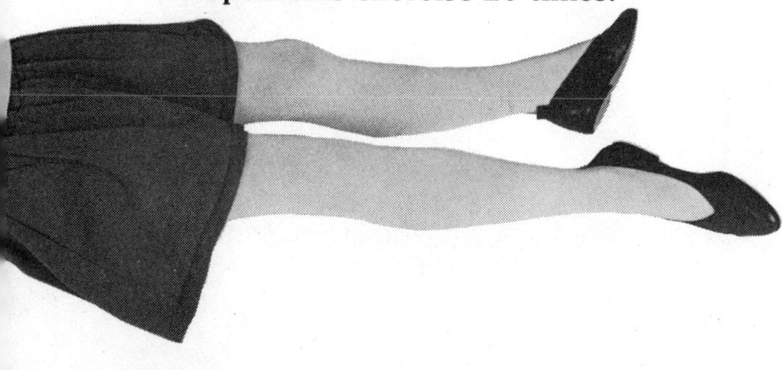

EXERCISE 2
OPEN WIDE

1. Still lying on your back in a relaxed position with your hands in place, breathe in through your mouth instead of your nose. Make sure you breathe slowly. Mouth breathing allows you to take in a greater amount of air rapidly, but if you breathe *too* rapidly, you may hyperventilate. If you begin to feel dizzy, slow down.

2. Hold your breath for a count of five. (None of these exercises need to be precisely timed. Once you've counted through them a few times, your body will remember the rhythms closely enough.)

3. Let the breath out slowly through your mouth to the count of ten, keeping the flow as even as you can. Think of your exhalation as a wave breaking gently along the beach, slowly rolling out along the sand.

4. Repeat this 20 times. Then move on to the next exercise.

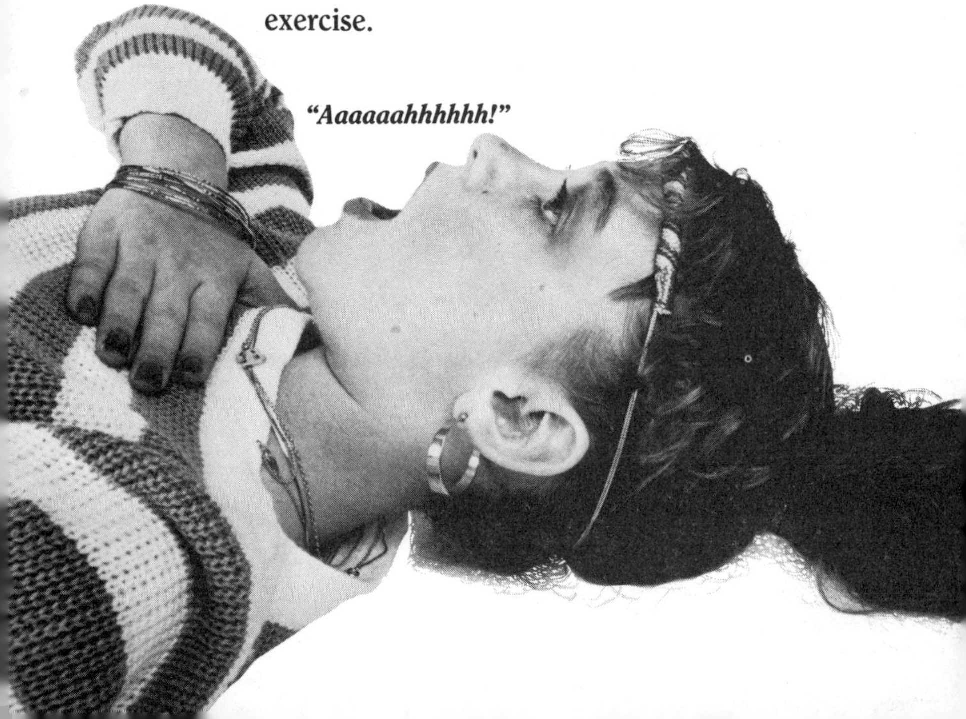

"Aaaaaahhhhhh!"

EXERCISE 3
SOUND OFF

Once you've got the proper rhythm, you can add sound. Remain in your relaxed position.

1. Repeat the mouth breathing, but this time instead of silently expelling your breath for a count of ten, make the vowel sound *ah,* drawn out over the entire exhalation: *aaaaaahhhhhh.* You should be able to feel the vibrations in your abdominal area. Don't be afraid to exaggerate the sound and the opening of your mouth. What you're practicing here is the coordination of your breathing with your speaking.

2. Now try this exercise with some other vowel sounds, for example:

ee (as in *freaking*)
ih (as in *bitchen*)
eh (as in *Melvin*)
ah (as in *max*)
aw (as in *awesome*)
uh (as in *vicious*)
o (as in *grody*)
oo (as in *bufu*)

3. When you've mastered the technique lying down, you can try it in the sitting and standing positions you are in when you do most of your speaking. Keep your hands on your upper chest and abdomen so that you can feel where you're breathing from.

4. Repeat each of the different vowel sounds five times.

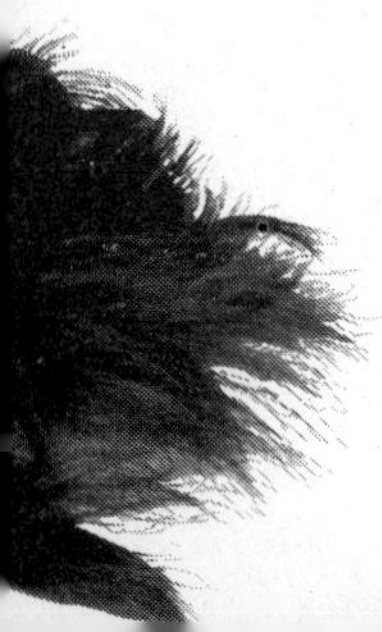

EXERCISE 4
SQUEEZE BOX

Most Valspeakers don't speak loudly enough, and one of the reasons is that there is simply not enough breath behind their words to get them out. If this is one of your problems, you can practice increasing your volume. Likewise, many Vals talk at too high a pitch, giving their communication a strident, little-girl sound. There is no single pitch that is appropriate for everyone, but you can use this technique to find your most natural one.

1. Remaining on your back in your relaxed position, place both your hands on your abdominal area.

2. Pressing down gently but continuously, make each of the vowel sounds used in *Sound Off.* The harder you push with your hands, the louder will be the sound that emerges.

3. Repeat each vowel sound at least three times before moving on to the next step.

4. Now, locate the pitch that is best for you. Take a breath through your mouth and as you exhale, say "uh-huh," as if you were agreeing with someone. Hold the *huh* and gently press your abdomen. The tone that you produce with this relaxed *huh* will be the one that is most comfortable and natural for you, and the one you should aim to produce in most of your speech.

5. Repeat this a few times or until you are sure the sound you are producing is comfortable for you.

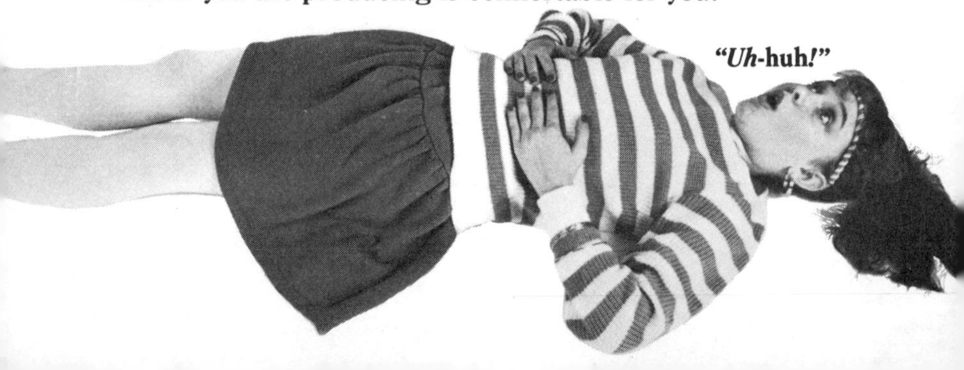

EXERCISE 5
BOOK CHAT

Breathing is also an important factor in the rapid-fire delivery that so many Valspeakers have. A breathing exercise to help control this tendency is simply to read aloud from one of your favorite books.

1. Sit up comfortably in chair in a quiet room with no distractions. Don't allow your body to slide into a slumped position while you read.

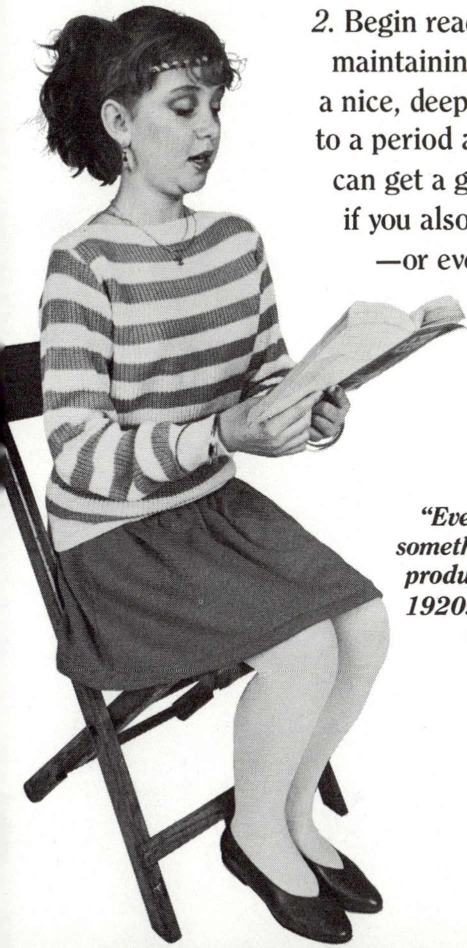

2. Begin reading aloud, concentrating on maintaining a slow, even pace. Stop for a nice, deep breath every time you come to a period at the end of a sentence. You can get a great deal out of this exercise if you also make a point of enunciating—or even exaggerating—each of the words in a sentence.

3. Continue reading aloud for at least five minutes a session.

"Every twenty years, it seems, something happens in America that produces a new strain of youth. In the 1920s we had the Flapper. Her hair was bobbed, . . . "

VOICE BOX

The larynx, commonly known as the voice box, is responsible for the musical and tonal qualities of your voice. The voice box takes the raw air moving up from the lungs and shapes it into the beginnings of intelligible speech.

One of the attributes of the voice that the larynx determines is the pitch. In the previous section we've seen how a breathing exercise can be used to find the optimum pitch for your speech. But once you've found that pitch, you don't want to use it for every word. That would be the vocal equivalent of finding one outfit and wearing it day after day, night after night—to school, to parties, and to bed. Variations in tone give your speech the same interest that variations in outfits lend to your wardrobe—and they are far cheaper.

EXERCISE 6
UPS AND DOWNS

The deadly Valley monotone can be eliminated by varying the stress given to different words or sounds. Stress is nothing more than making certain sounds more prominent than those surrounding them. It can be achieved by making them higher or lower in pitch, by making them louder, or by increasing their duration (as in "*sooooo* grody"). A simple exercise for varying the pitch of your voice is to take the same vowel sounds you used in your breathing exercises and glide up and down the scale with them.

1. Sit up straight in a comfortable chair. Pretend there is a string attached to the top of your head pulling you up. Take a deep breath through your mouth, and starting with the lowest note you can make say the sound *ee*. Glide the sound up the scale, stop briefly at the highest note, then glide down to the note you began with.

2. Repeat the *ee* sound ten times.

3. Repeat each of the following vowel sounds ten times each, gliding from the lowest note you can make to the highest, then back down: *ih, eh, ah, aw, uh, oh, oo.*

4. Once you have the hang of the glide, try doing the same thing with two-syllable words: *Mel* (up)–*vin* (down), *gro* (up)–*dy* (down), *awe* (up)–*some* (down).

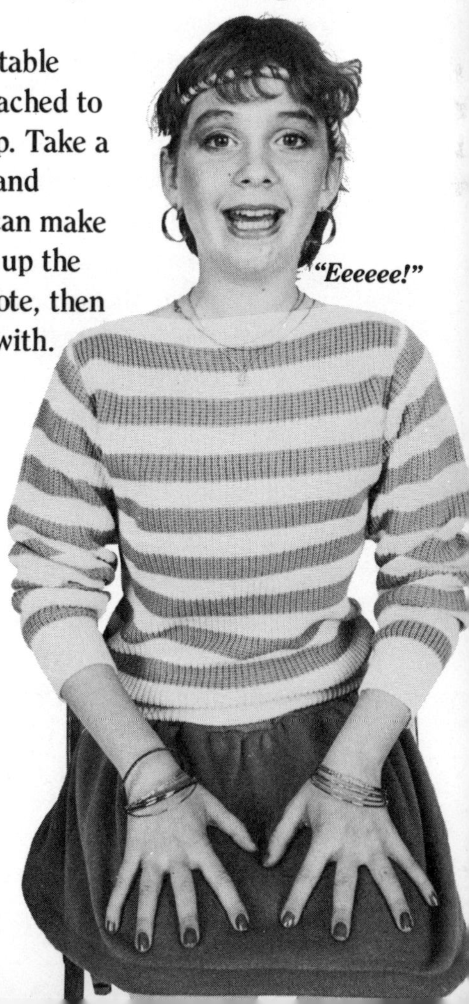

"Eeeeee!"

EXERCISE 7
SEESAW SENTENCES

Once you've gotten the feel of raising and lowering pitch with these words, you can apply the principle to whole sentences. For these purposes, the Valley vocabulary is as good as any other. If you have any trouble varying the pitch of these words, a piano or guitar may be helpful. Find a note that is comfortable for your voice and sing the first syllable; then use a neighboring note (higher or lower) for the next syllable.

1. Remain seated in your comfortable chair. Keep your back straight and head up. Take a breath and say the following sentences, being sure to raise the pitch on the last word of each:

Grody to the *max* (up)
Barf me *out* (up)
Gag me with a *spoon* (up)

2. Repeat each sentence ten times.

3. Now say the same phrases, only this time drop the pitch on the last word of each:

Grody to the *max* (down)
Barf me *out* (down)
Gag me with a *spoon* (down)

4. Repeat each sentence ten times.

5. Finally, try raising and lowering the pitch of alternating syllables within each phrase:

Gro (up)–*dy* (down) *to* (up) *the* (down) *max* (up)
Barf (down) *me* (up) *out* (down)
Gag (up) *me* (down) *with* (up) *a* (down) *spoon* (up)

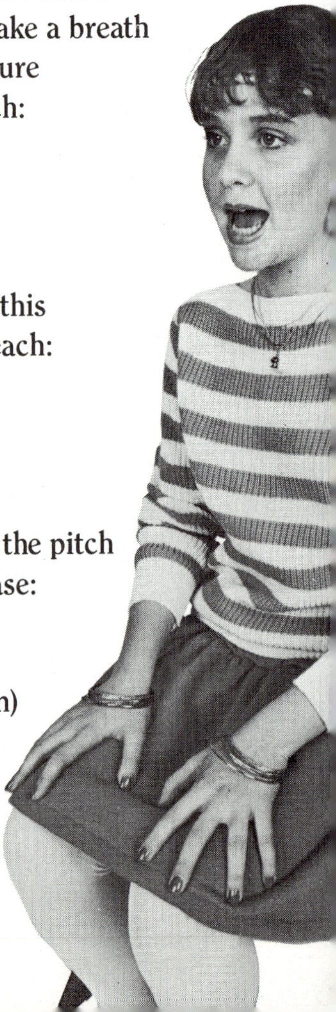

EXERCISE 8
LOUD AND CLEAR

The next way to stress words is to make them louder. Much Valley talk is so dull because it is not only delivered at the same pitch, but also at the same intensity—not very intense. A simple test to determine if you are speaking loudly enough (besides counting how many times your parents ask you to speak up) involves the use of your cassette deck. Most of these have meters that show the strength of the signal being recorded—either a needle that registers in a certain range (usually marked in red) when the volume level is optimal, or maybe a row of blinking lights.

1. Making sure the room is quiet, stand about an arm's length away from the microphone. Make sure you can see the sound meter. Recite a few of the sentences from the previous exercise. You should be able to tell visually whether or not you're projecting enough sound.

2. Without changing the volume control on your recorder, stand the same distance away from the mike and record your own voice.

3. Play back the tape. Be aware of fading out at the end of your sentences, a typical Valley problem that should be corrected.

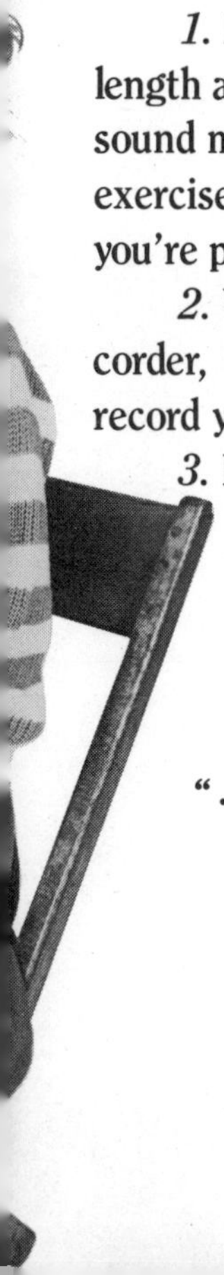

"**. . . *to the* max.**"

EXERCISE 9
STEPPING STONES

The same voice level tests can be a help in another volume exercise.

1. Say the phrases from the previous exercises, but this time emphasize each word successively by making it louder than the rest of the phrase:

Grody to the max
Grody *to* the max
Grody to *the* max
Grody to the *max*

2. Do this with each of the other phrases, or with any others that are fun to say.

EXERCISE 10
THE SYLLABLE STRETCH

You can also improve the stress you put on words by doing a similar exercise that focuses on the *duration* of words, stretching out different ones.

1. Really exaggerate one syllable in each short sentence. For example:

Baaaaaarrrrrrffffff me out
Barf *meeeeee* out
Barf me *ouuuuuut*

2. Repeat this sentence ten times; then move on to the next.

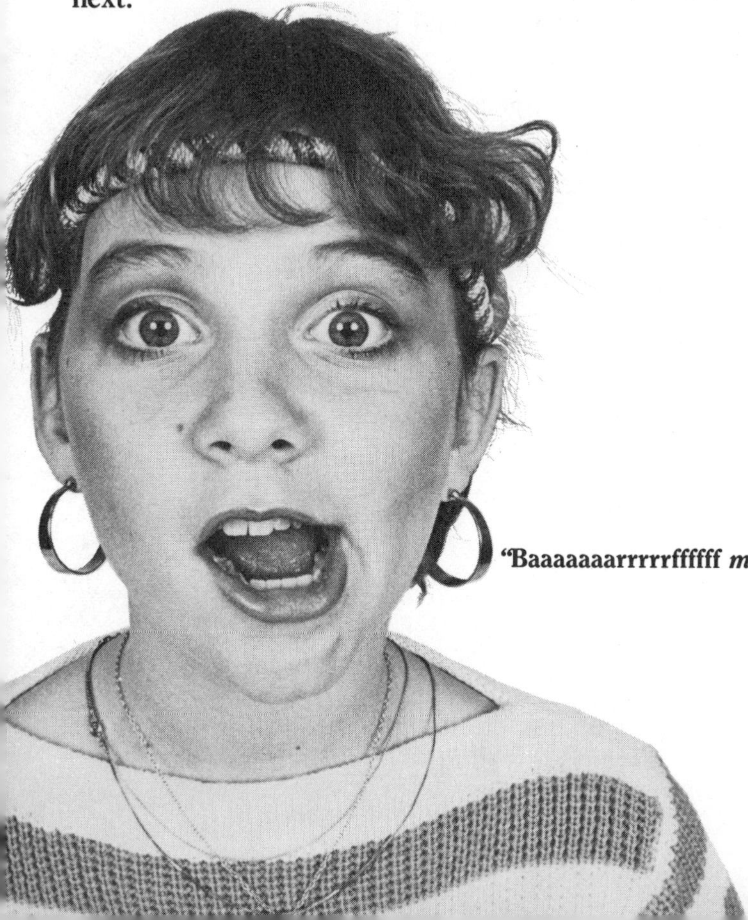

"Baaaaaaarrrrrffffff *me out!*"

ARTICULATION

No matter how beautiful the quality of your voice and the music of your speech, if your words can't be understood, you might as well save your breath. Most Valley speakers have perfectly developed articulatory apparatus; they're just too insecure or lazy to use it. They seem to aspire toward the ventriloquist's lack of mouth movement, although instead of throwing their voices out toward their audience, they throw their voices in. Unfortunately, there's nobody down there to hear them.

One result of this lack of mouth movement is that most Valspeak vowel sounds tend toward the middle of the vowel scale. "Really" gets lowered toward the middle so that it comes out "rilly," while a low-range vowel sound like "fully" gets raised so that it comes out "filly."

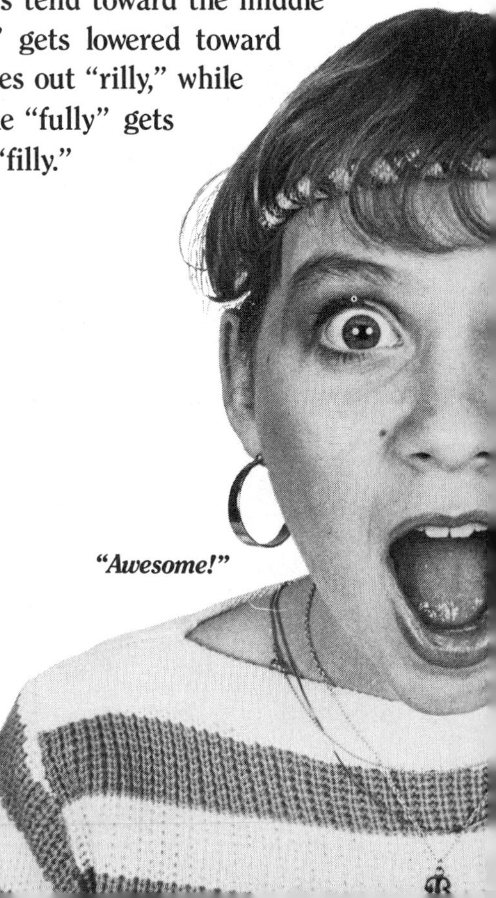

"Awesome!"

EXERCISE 11
JAWING

If articulation is one of your problems, this exercise will get your mouth moving.

1. Sit up straight in a comfortable chair. Practice a kind of exaggerated yawning or chewing motion by letting your jaw drop as you go through the same vowel sounds you worked with in the breathing exercise. They will sound like this: *yee, yih, yeh, yah, yaw, yuh, yo, yoo.*

2. Repeat this series straight through ten times, trying to feel the hinging in your jaw.

3. Now try running through the gamut of vowel sounds, using whole words from the Valspeak vocabulary:

ee: beastie, really, mini, tweeked
ih: billies, pig out, vicious, wicked
eh: Melvin, mega
ah: jazzed, gag me, thrashed, radical, max
aw: awesome
uh: vicious
o: gross, grody, Lowies
oo: bufu, goober, with a spoon

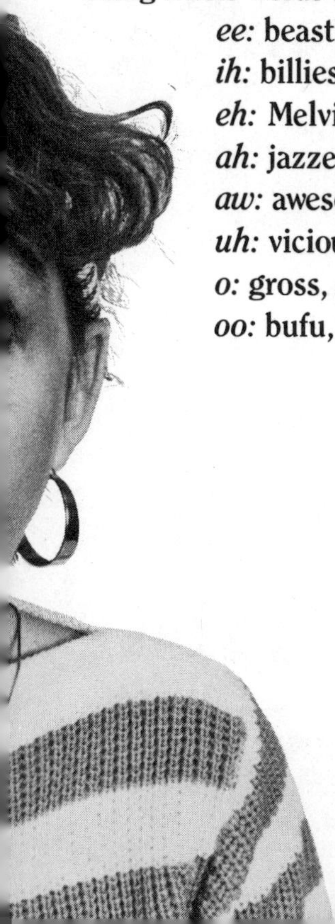

EXERCISE 12
SIS BOOM GLIDE

You can also use Valley words to practice articulation of the consonant sounds. Of these, the most difficult for habitual Valspeakers are the plosives: the sounds of the letters *p, b, t, d, k,* and *g.* They require energy to produce their little explosions of air.

1. Sitting up straight in a comfortable chair (keep your head up), practice each of the plosive sounds by putting them at the beginning of the vowel sounds shown in the previous exercise: *tee, tih, teh, tah, taw, toe, too.*

2. Now try the same thing with the plosive sounds in the middle position, between the vowel sounds: *eeTee, ihTih, ehTeh, ahTah, awTaw, uhTuh, oToe, ooToo.*

3. Finally, place the plosive sounds at the end of each vowel sound: *eeT, ihT, ehT, ahT, awT, uhT, oaT, ooT.*

4. Do this exercise with the *p, b, d, k,* and *g* sounds as well as the *t.* Try to draw out the vowel sound and make the plosive as crisp and sharp as you can. If you have a feather, hold it in front of your lips. If it moves, you can be sure the air is puffing out.

5. Now do this exercise with the fricative sounds, *s, z, ch, sh, zh, f, v,* and *th.*

6. Finally, practice the vowel sounds using the glides, *l* and *r.*

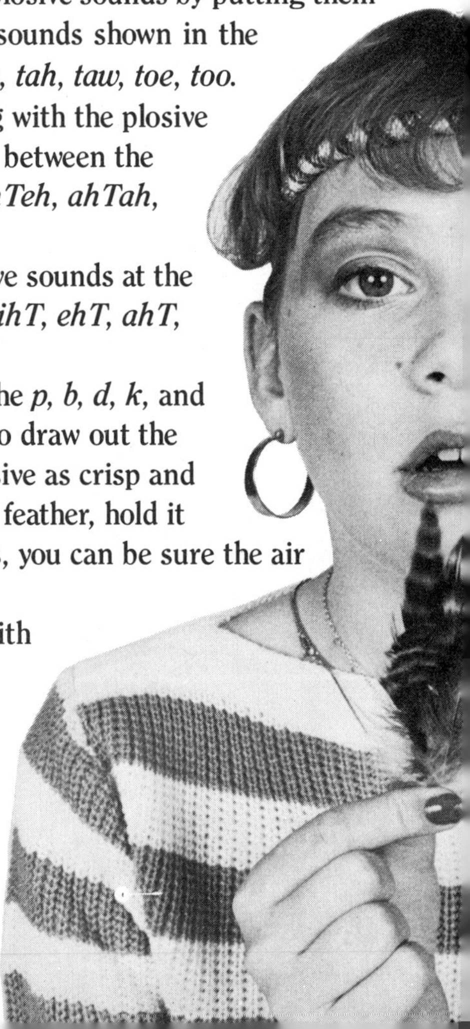

EXERCISE 13
ADVANCED SIS BOOM GLIDE

For a more advanced form of the same exercise, try using whole sentences of Valley words, putting the plosive, fricative, and glide sounds in the beginning, middle, and ends of them. You will note that in this and the following exercise, English equivalents are provided under each Valspeak sentence for the bilingual.

1. Begin with the plosives:

*Bobby is a b*itchen *b*a*b*e.
Ro*b* is undenia*b*ly *b*eautiful.

An*d*rea *d*ate*d* a nur*d*.
An*d*rea was escorte*d* by a *d*un*d*erhea*d*.

Ba*g* your face, you me*g*a-*g*oober.
Be*g*one, you bi*g g*oon.

*K*elly frea*k*ed out the gee*k*.
*K*elly drove the tac*k*y jer*k* crazy.

Patricia, a *p*re*pp*ie, threw u*p*.
Patrick, an u*pp*er-class twer*p*, regurgitated.

The *t*o*t*al beas*t*ie pigged ou*t*.
The *t*erribly una*tt*rac*t*ive ci*t*izen overa*t*e.

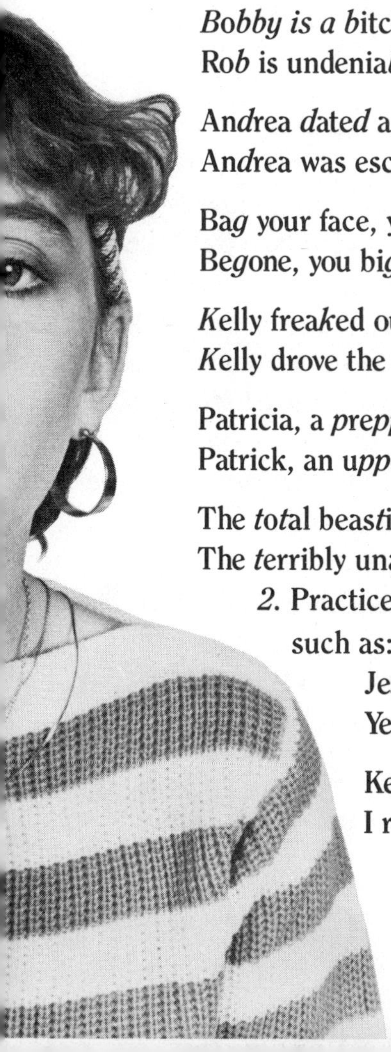

2. Practice the fricative sounds in sentences such as:

Je*ss*ie is *s*ooooo gro*ss*.
Ye*s*, Je*ss*ie is certainly di*s*gu*s*ting.

Ke*v*in is my fa*v*e *v*iciou*s* Dude.
I ra*v*e *v*ery *v*ociferou*s*ly o*v*er Ke*v*in.

He is a *f*ully bu*f* sur*f*er.
He looks *f*ine even a*f*ter *f*alling o*ff* a sur*f*board.

3. Now apply this technique to the glide sounds. You can use the following sentences or make up your own:

Che*ryl* has the bi*ll*ies for some *L*owies.
Che*ryl* has the *l*ega*l* tende*r* for the *l*age*r*.

The su*r*f is *r*ea*ll*y tubula*r*.
The *r*ipp*l*es a*r*e exquisite*l*y fo*r*med.

EXERCISE 14
NOSE NO-NO'S

One of the biggest problems of Valspeakers is excessive nasality. Like so many other difficulties, it arises partly from the Val's reluctance to open her mouth. In normal English, there are some sounds that are *supposed* to be nasal—the *m*, *n*, and *ng* sounds.

1. Sitting up straight in a comfortable chair (head up, too), first check to see if you are saying the above sounds correctly. Hold the bridge of your nose gently between your thumb and forefinger. Say the *m* sound, exaggerating it slightly—*mmmmmm*. If you feel a little vibration when you make the sound, you are producing it nasally.

2. Repeat this for the *n* and *ng* sounds.

3. Try the following sentences. You should feel the vibration of nasality:

O*m*igod, it's aweso*m*e to the *m*ax.
*M*ercy *m*e, it's a*m*azi*ng*ly *m*arvelous.

Shi*n*e that *m*ajor ska*n*ky ho*n*ker.
Sta*n*d up that *n*otoriously ob*n*oxious perso*n*.

4. Now try the following sentences. You should feel no vibration. If you do feel vibration, open your mouth until it disappears:

He's really way hyper.
He's very excited.

The dude is totally buf.
That fellow is truly attractive.

5. Repeat the non-nasal sentences ten times each, keeping your thumb and forefinger on the bridge of your nose to check for vibrations.

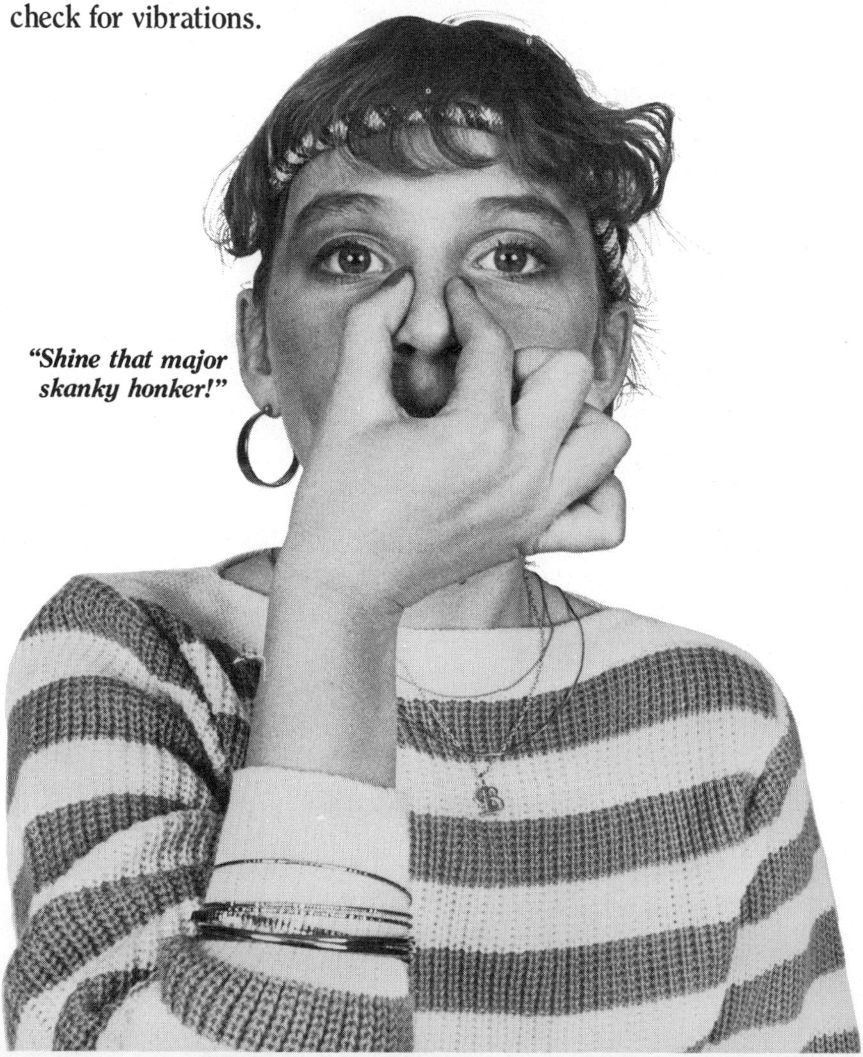

"Shine that major skanky honker!"

VOCAL IMAGE

Exercises in breathing, stress, and articulation may give the impression that speaking is a strictly mechanical process that can be changed by strictly mechanical techniques. In fact, what you say and how you say it is determined as much by psychological factors as by physical ones.

To the Greek philosopher Galen, speech was the mirror of the soul. You can train yourself to stress any word in any sentence, but which words do you actually stress in conversation? What do mumbled speech or machine-gun delivery tell people about your self-confidence and anxiety levels?

If you have access to a videotape camera and playback machine, you have a powerful tool for deprogramming your Valley habits. Equally useful and more accessible, a full-length mirror can also give you an accurate reflection of how you're coming off. By actually seeing and hearing yourself as others do, you can become aware of—and change—any mannerisms that gross you out.

EXERCISE 15

FROM THE GUTS

The simplest and most effective exercise you can do to improve your vocal image is to practice talking about how you really feel.

1. Sit comfortably in front of your mirror (or video camera). Maintaining eye contact with yourself during your entire talk, and without using excessive movement, recount the events of the day. For example:

> What did you experience when you got back a grade on a test in school?
>
> How did you react when a friend ignored you?
>
> How did you feel when your parents scolded or praised you?

2. Carefully note your image. Are your eyes wandering all over the place? Try to direct them back to establish eye contact. Is your head and body bobbing and flopping when you talk? Concentrate on keeping movement to a minimum—it is difficult to pay attention to someone who bobs while she talks.

3. Practice this exercise, concentrating on a different aspect of your image each session. Soon you will see and hear someone much easier to listen to.

EXERCISE 16
ACTING OUT

Once you have controlled aimless eye, head, and body movements, begin working on getting your movements to work for you. They can help communicate what you are saying.

1. Stand comfortably in front of your full-length mirror. Describe yourself as being *thrashed.* Let your shoulders slump, show the fatigue in your eyes—look really tired.

2. Now describe yourself as being *jazzed.* Look animated—let your face and your posture express excitement.

3. Describe yourself as *totally grossed out.* See the disgust in your face and in your body movements.

4. Now try turning off the sound. Just express the various emotions without describing them.

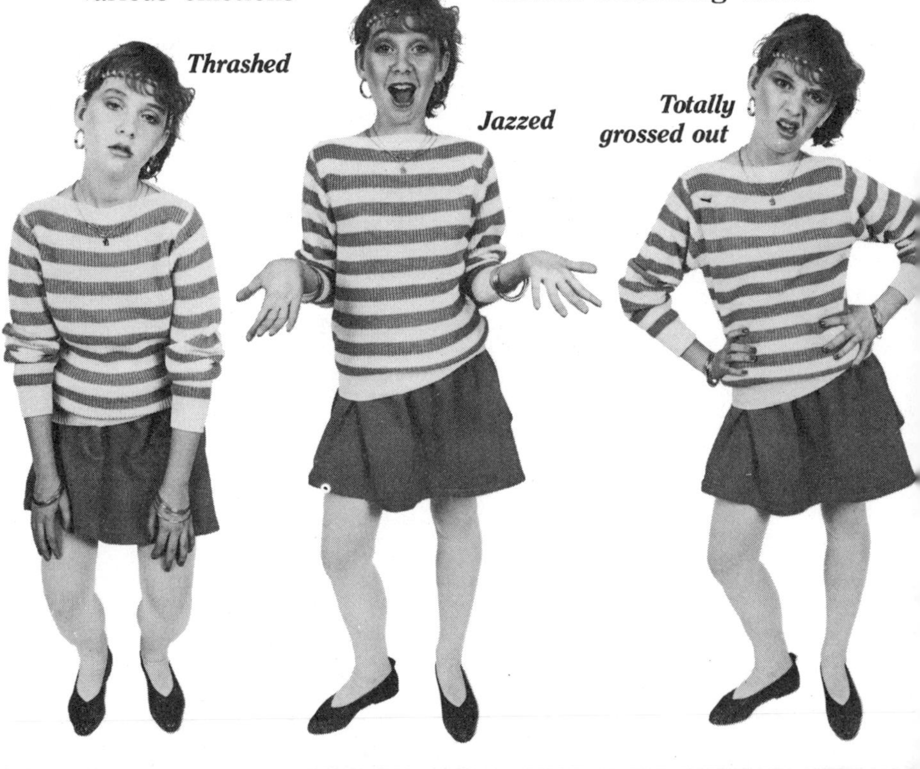

EXERCISE 17
TURNING OUT

Turning out is not really an exercise—it's a final reminder. Just as important as developing the skills to make yourself understood is developing the ability to listen to others. Practice turning your attention outward by paying attention to what others are saying. Watch their expressions and listen to the music of their speech. Hear not only *what* they say, but *how* they say it.

NOTE: If you'd like to work more closely with a speech-language pathologist in your area, give the National Association for Hearing and Speech Action a call (collect) at (301) 897-8682, or write to their headquarters at The Public Information Office, NAHSA, 10801 Rockville Pike, Rockville, Maryland 20852. They will send you a list of certified professionals in your area—fer shurr!